Report of The Commission on Nursing

A blueprint for the future

ISBN 0-7076-6122-6

BAILE ÁTHA CLIATH

ARNA FHOILSIÚ AG OIFIG AN tSOLÁTHAIR

Le ceannach díreach ón

OIFIG DHÍOLTA FOILSEACHÁN RIALTAIS,

TEACH SUN ALLIANCE, SRÁID THEACH LAIGHEAN, BAILE ÁTHA CLIATH 2,

nó tríd an bpost ó

FOILSEACHÁIN RIALTAIS, AN RANNÓG POST-TRÁCHTA,

4 - 5 BÓTHAR FHEARCHAIR, BAILE ÁTHA CLIATH 2,

(Teil: 01-6613111 - fo-líne 4040/4045; Fax: 01-4752760)

nó trí aon díoltóir leabhar.

DUBLIN

PUBLISHED BY THE STATIONERY OFFICE

To be purchased directly from the

GOVERNMENT PUBLICATIONS SALE OFFICE,

SUN ALLIANCE HOUSE, MOLESWORTH STREET, DUBLIN 2,

or by mail order from

GOVERNMENT PUBLICATIONS, POSTAL TRADE SECTION,

4 - 5 HARCOURT ROAD, DUBLIN 2,

(Tel: 01-6613111 - ext. 4040/4045; Fax: 01-4752760)

or through any bookseller.

£12.00

Commission on Nursing

21 Fitzwilliam Square, Dublin 2.
Phone: (01) 676 3837 Fax: (01) 676 3847

31 July 1998

Mr. Brian Cowen, T.D.
Minister for Health and Children
Department of Health and
Children
Hawkins House
Dublin 2

Dear Minister,

I have the honour to submit to you, on behalf of the Commission on Nursing, our final report which we have prepared in accordance with the terms of reference given to us.

Mella Carroll

Ms. Justice Mella Carroll
Chair of the
Commission on Nursing

Contents

Glossary of Terms

Accreditation

Process by which a statutory or professional body certifies and recognises an educational course as meeting the requirements for professional recognition.

Active File

A file of nurses on the register who are not on the inactive file.

An Bord Altranais

The Nursing Board (referred to as "the Board" in the report) is the statutory regulatory body for nursing and midwifery established under the Nurses Act 1985.

Blue Book

The findings of the Adjudications Tribunal issued on September 23rd, 1996, being revised proposals for agreement on the pay and conditions of nurses referred to in the Labour Court recommendation LCR 15450, dated 7th March 1997.

Candidate Register

A register, maintained by the Board, of students admitted for training in the disciplines of general, sick children's, mental handicap, midwifery and psychiatry.

Category II Approval

Approval given by the Board to post-registration courses designed, developed and conducted with reference to a specific body of knowledge and experience in an area of nursing, which meet criteria set by the Board.

Department of Health

Title changed to Department of Health and Children on 12 July 1997.

Discipline

Discipline in the Irish context refers to the branches of nursing which are registerable with the Board, namely general, psychiatry, mental handicap, midwifery, sick children's, public health nursing and nurse tutors.

Division

The register of nurses maintained by the Board is divided into seven divisions named after the disciplines as detailed above.

Inactive File

The Board maintains an inactive file of nurses on the register who are not practising nursing in Ireland.

Minister for Health

Title changed to Minister for Health and Children on 12 July 1997 (referred to as "the Minister" in the report).

Nursing Alliance

The coalition of the four nursing unions - Irish Nurses Organisation, Psychiatric Nurses Association, SIPTU and IMPACT.

Register

The register of nurses maintained by the Board pursuant to the Nurses Act 1985.

Supernumerary

Not included in the rostered complement of nurses or midwives.

Validation

Pathway or course approval process used in higher education. A panel of academic staff scrutinises the curriculum and challenge the pathway team on their curriculum design.

Executive Summary and Summary of the Main Recommendations

Nursing and midwifery have been one of the cornerstones of the modern Irish health service. The quality of care and public satisfaction with the health service is often related to the quality of the nursing service. Irish nurses not only enjoy the confidence of patients and clients of the health service but have an international reputation for their professionalism and the excellence of their care. However, the health services are in a state of constant and rapid development in response to technological, social and economic changes both domestically and internationally. The Commission is recommending a new framework which will give a secure basis for the further professional development of nursing and midwifery in the context of anticipated changes in the health services, their organisation and delivery.

The Nurses Act 1985 provides the current statutory framework for the regulation of the profession. It provided for the establishment of An Bord Altranais or the Nursing Board (the Board) to oversee the regulation of the profession. The Board has a membership of twenty nine, seventeen of whom are elected by the profession and twelve of whom are appointed by the Minister for Health and Children (the Minister). The Commission considers that there is a need for the profession to take greater responsibility for its own regulation and practice and that the Board needs to undertake a more pro-active professional leadership role whilst ensuring the protection of the public. There is also the need to give the Board a more distinctly independent identity from the Department of Health and Children and the nursing trade unions. The Commission has recommended a revised membership of the Board composed of elected members of the profession together with three persons to represent the public interest appointed by the Minister. The Board would also have the option of nominating up to four persons from specified categories, to be appointed by the Minister.

The fitness to practise procedures were criticised during the consultative process as being inflexible and excessively legalistic at all stages of an inquiry. The Commission reviewed fitness to practise procedures for other professions in Ireland and the procedures operated by the United Kingdom Central Council for Nursing, Midwifery and Health Visiting. The Commission recommends a more flexible fitness to practise procedure which will allow for an early review of a complaint and for a subsequent differentiation between an issue arising as a consequence of the health of a nurse or midwife or as a consequence of misconduct.

Midwives, during the consultative process, stated that the current regulatory framework did not sufficiently recognise their distinct identity and concerns. The Commission considers that midwifery has a distinct focus relating to the care of women during pregnancy and following birth, which differentiates it from nursing. Therefore, the Commission has recommended the establishment of a statutory midwives committee within the Board which will be responsible for issues relating to the scope of practice in midwifery.

It was suggested during the consultative process that the Board should take responsibility for the regulation of care assistants and other non-nursing personnel. The Commission does not consider that the Board should take on this role and considers the control of care assistants and non-nursing personnel as essentially a matter for employers. There is a need for the Department of Health and Children, health service providers and nursing organisations to establish standardised criteria in relation to entry requirements, education qualifications and training for such personnel across the health service.

Nurses and midwives are currently providing an excellent service in sometimes difficult circumstances. The rapidly changing pace of the health service is placing increasing demands and expectations on the profession. The Commission, in considering the future needs of the health service and international developments in preparation for the profession, was of the view that there was a need to examine the pre-registration education of nurses. The Commission considered that members of the profession in the future would be required to possess increased flexibility and the ability to work autonomously. The future health service will also require greater inter-disciplinary co-operation in the delivery of health care. In order to meet expected future needs the Commission has recommended that pre-registration nursing education be based on a four year degree programme, incorporating one year of employment, with structured clinical placement in the health service and be fully integrated within the third-level education sector. The recommended change in the educational qualification of nurses on registration will not impact on the professional status of existing registered nurses. This is evidenced by experience in other countries such as Australia and other professions which have moved from apprenticeship schemes to third-level degree programmes. The transition will require careful planning and a forum of interested parties should be established to agree a strategy for the implementation of the pre-registration nursing degree programme. The transition to a degree programme should take place at the start of the academic year in 2002.

The Commission recognises the invaluable contribution of nurse educators to the high quality and international standing of Irish nurses. The proposed changes in the pre-registration education of nurses will have a major impact on the future role of nurse educators. The Commission recommends that health service employers undertake a detailed consultation with each nurse tutor currently involved in the pre-registration education of nurses to determine their desired future career pathway. Such pathways may involve either a move into third-level institutes, other educational avenues in continuing education or a pathway in management or clinical practice. Health service providers should support nurse tutors in upgrading their educational or other qualifications to facilitate their transition to their desired career pathway. Many nurse tutors will be able to transfer into third-level institutes within the academic career pathway. However, some nurse tutors may not have had opportunities to carry out the research or publish the material expected of those entering an academic career pathway within the third-level sector. In order to facilitate the transfer of as many nurse tutors as possible to the third-level sector, the Commission recommends the creation of "nurse lecturer" posts within third-level institutes. Such posts would retain the same salary and conditions of nurse tutors and appointments would be made on a personal basis to the individual nurse tutor. The Commission also recommends that joint appointments take place between third-level institutes and health service providers. Schools of nursing will in future become centres of nursing education providing educational and training resources to nurses working in the health services.

The consultative process identified an increasing demand for and proliferation of post-registration education for the profession. In addition, the absence of a clinical career pathway in nursing and midwifery was seen as increasingly limiting the development of the profession. The Commission recommends the establishment of a National Council for the Professional Development of Nursing and Midwifery (the National Council) to give guidance and direction in relation to the development of specialist nursing and midwifery posts and post-registration educational programmes offered to nurses and midwives. The National Council will be an independent statutory body with its own officers and will administer its own budget. The National Council will work closely with the Board and will not accredit courses, if in the view of the Board, the practice outcomes of a proposed course are not within the parameters of professional standards and scope of practice guidelines. It will have a board of twenty members appointed by the Minister for a five year period. A large component of the work of the proposed National Council will be to bring a coherent approach to the progression of specialisation and the development of a clinical career pathway for nursing and midwifery. The Commission recommends the development of a three step clinical career pathway by the creation of clinical nurse or midwife specialist (CNS) posts and advanced nurse or midwife practitioner (ANP) posts. The recognition of CNS or ANP status must be matched with specific posts within the health service. Those with CNS or ANP status will be characterised by extensive relevant experience, appropriate post-registration educational qualifications and an extended scope of practice. The development of specialisms and post-registration education programmes will be overseen by the National Council. It is important that there is coherence and equity of access to the necessary post-registration educational programmes. Interim arrangements will apply for the appointment of an initial cohort of CNSs and ANPs.

The Commission is conscious that many excellent nurses and midwives, who will remain primarily responsible for the delivery of high quality care, may not wish to specialise and seek promotion. It was suggested that there needed to be increased recognition for these senior staff nurses and midwives. The Commission recommends that the question of additional recognition for long service for staff nurses and midwives should be examined through established structures. Also outstanding claims for allowances should be referred to the Labour Court as a matter of urgency.

The Commission attaches particular importance to the development of nursing and midwifery research at every level; within each individual organisation (hospital or community), at health board level and within the Department of Health and Children. If nursing and midwifery practice is to be evidence-based, research should form an integral part of all aspects of nursing and midwifery. However, there is a need to ensure that nursing and midwifery research is seen within the context of the overall research activity of the health service and maintains a high level of quality. The Commission recommends that the Minister provides for nursing and midwifery research to be funded through the Health Research Board, makes funding available specifically for nursing and midwifery research and appoints a registered nurse or midwife with experience in research to the Health Research Board. A nursing and midwifery research advisory division should be established within the Health Research Board.

A range of issues was raised during the consultative process in relation to the role of nurses and midwives in the management of services. These concerns included the need for greater internal communication within organisations, a need for the greater involvement of nurses and midwives in planning and policy development, a concern that nursing and midwifery management was preoccupied with hierarchies and the detailed control of nurses and midwives, rather than the management of the professional function and the related need for the greater devolution of authority within the nursing and midwifery management structure.

The development of an effective internal communication system is essential to the on-going effectiveness and success of an organisation. Such systems need to be audited on an on-going basis to ensure their continuing effectiveness in conveying and receiving information.

The Commission recommends the further development of the post of Chief Nursing Officer within the Department of Health and Children. The Commission also recommends the establishment of a Nursing and Midwifery Planning and Development Unit within each health board. Such units will have a range of responsibilities and will bring a greater focus and coherence to the development and quality assurance of nursing and midwifery within each health board.

Structural reforms within nursing and midwifery management are required. There needs to be greater devolution of authority to nursing and midwifery management at the unit of care level. Senior nursing and midwifery management should focus to a much greater extent on strategic planning and quality assurance. Middle nursing management needs to be given clearly delegated responsibility such as in the management of an area of care or designated functional responsibilities. The Commission considers first line nursing management as essential to the effective operation and on-going development of a high quality health service. First line nursing and midwifery managers have to balance management skills with clinical credibility. Clerical support and information technology should be made available to first line nursing and midwifery management, where appropriate. The Commission recommends the development of first line nursing and midwifery management to fulfil the functions of professional leadership, staffing and staff development, resource management and facilitating communication. The title of first line nursing and midwifery management should be changed to clinical nurse manager or clinical midwife manager. Given the crucial role of first line nursing and midwifery management and the complexity and activity level of certain areas of the health service, the Commission considers that there is scope for three grades of first line nursing and midwifery management. All three grades would rarely be in place in a single unit and only one person would be designated as being in overall charge of a single unit of care or ward. The three grades would be clinical nurse manager 1 or clinical midwife manager 1, clinical nurse manager 2 or clinical midwife manager 2, or clinical nurse manager 3 or clinical midwife manager 3.

The development of future nurse and midwife managers should be supported to a greater extent. A number of issues which impact on the personnel management of nursing and midwifery and the work environment are identified and will require an enlightened management approach for the well-being of the work force. Low morale, such as was caused by an excessive amount of temporary employment, should not be allowed to recur.

There is also a need for a long-term financial commitment to developing communication, management information and support systems to allow for greater devolution of budgets and staff development programmes. These programmes should be underpinned by the allocation of adequate resources and a commitment to on-going funding.

Particular concerns in relation to nursing in the community were raised during the consultative process. An increasing number of groups are now providing nursing and midwifery services in the community and there were concerns in relation to the future direction and integration of these services. There appears to be little consensus within the profession in relation to the future direction of nursing and midwifery in the community. The Commission recommends the development of public health nursing and recommends that the Department of Health and Children issue a revised strategy statement on the role of public health nursing. The strategy statement will replace the Department of Health circular which issued in 1966 and is still seen as the basis of the public health nursing service. The Commission recommends the continuation of the present area-based model of public health nursing. However, public health nurses should be allowed focus to a greater extent on a health promotion and preventive role in the community. In light of the range of services offered by public health nurses, the Commission considers that registration as a midwife should no longer be a mandatory requirement for entry to the higher diploma in public health nursing or registration as a public health nurse.

There is a need to refocus management responsibilities within public health nursing. The superintendent public health nurse should play a greater strategic and clinical leadership role whilst delegating greater responsibility for operational issues to the senior public health nurse. The on-going development of public health nursing will also entail a permanent role for registered general nurses in the community care nursing team in line with service need. The Commission also recommends the development of mental handicap and psychiatric nursing services in the community. The development of clinical nurse specialists and advanced practitioners within these services should enhance the delivery of nursing services in the community. The Commission also recommends a framework to assist the professional development of practice nurses working in general practices.

Care of the elderly is an increasingly important area of nursing activity. It offers opportunities for the development of nurse led services which will greatly enhance the services being delivered to patients and clients. There is a perception that nursing in care of the elderly is viewed in certain quarters as a "Cinderella" service. There were concerns in relation to conditions and staffing in care of the elderly. The Commission recommends that the Department of Health and Children examine, as a matter of urgency, conditions and staffing levels in care of the elderly services. The on-going development of nursing services in care of the elderly should also encompass the development of inter-disciplinary educational programmes and nursing services.

The Commission considered particular concerns relating to the disciplines of mental handicap nursing, midwifery and sick children's nursing. It appeared from the consultative process that mental handicap and sick children's nursing had a low profile amongst the public and within the profession. Midwifery had distinct concerns in relation to the education of midwives and the delivery of domiciliary midwifery services.

The Commission considers mental handicap nursing as essential to the delivery of a high quality service to clients with an intellectual disability. The Commission recommends that there is a need to promote the distinct identity and unique working environment of mental handicap nursing. Paediatric services are increasingly required to meet the needs of ever more acutely ill children. In view of developments within the service, the need for maturity in caring for children and traditional difficulties in recruiting students, the Commission recommends that sick children's nursing remain a post registration qualification. The content, duration and academic award for sick children's nursing should be reviewed in the light of the proposed move of pre-registration nursing education to degree level.

Concerns were expressed during the consultative process in relation to the current programme of education for midwifery, particularly in relation to the theoretical content of the programme. The Commission recommends that the Board review the current midwifery education programme as a matter of urgency. The supervision and regulation of domiciliary midwifery practice was the subject of much debate during the consultative process. There are currently fourteen independent domiciliary midwives practising in Ireland. The Commission considers that the determination of the suitability of midwives to provide an independent domiciliary service and the parameters of their practice are matters for the Board.

Issues relating to the retirement of nurses and midwives were raised during the consultative process. These included the equity of current provisions for the early retirement of psychiatric nurses which do not apply to other disciplines, problems with the pension entitlement of temporary nurses and nurses who have worked abroad for a number of years and the pension implications of flexible part-time working arrangements. The Commission referred these issues to the Commission on Public Service Pensions which is examining the occupational pension arrangements of public servants and is in a better position to examine these complex and difficult issues within the overall context of public service pensions.

The Commission was concerned at the reported level of bullying taking place at all levels of nursing and midwifery during the consultative process. The development of formal and informal procedures to deal with bullying in the workplace is recommended by the Commission.

The executive summary merely outlines the general framework proposed by the Commission for the development of the profession into the twenty-first century. The report details the rationale for the proposed framework and contains a range of detailed recommendations on related issues.

In relation to the implementation of the report, the Commission recommends that a monitoring committee be established which will issue yearly reports. It is envisaged that recommendations without a suggested time scale will be implemented as soon as practicable and in any event by the end of 2002. In addition to time scales identified in the report, there are four recommendations perceived as urgent: the forum (for pre-registration education), the National Council (for post-registration education), the Planning and Development Units in each health board, all of which should be established at the earliest possible date, and the legislation amending the Nurses Act 1985 which should be introduced before the Oireachtas by early 1999.

Main Recommendations on the Regulation of the Profession

- The Commission recommends that the nursing profession take greater responsibility for the regulation and practice of the profession and for ensuring professional leadership in nursing and midwifery. (4.2)

- The Commission recommends that the profession take greater control over its own destiny through ownership of the Board. (4.12)

- The Commission recommends section 6(1) of the 1985 Act be amended to provide that the general concern of the Board shall be the protection of the public through the promotion of high standards of professional education, training and practice and professional conduct among nurses and midwives. (4.13)

- The Commission recommends that section 51(2) of the 1985 Act be amended to provide that it shall be a function of the Board to give professional guidance and support on matters relating to clinical practice as well as giving guidance on all matters relating to ethical conduct and behaviour. (4.14)

- The Commission recommends that the 1985 Act be amended to provide that the Board shall consist of a maximum of 28 members appointed in the following way:

(a) eight nurses resident in the State, three of whom are representative of nurses engaged in clinical practice in general nursing (one of whom shall be working in care of the elderly), two of whom are representative of nurses engaged in clinical practice in psychiatric nursing and three of whom are nurses engaged in clinical practice in each of the following disciplines, sick children's, mental handicap and public health nursing, respectively, elected by nurses;

(b) five nurses resident in the State who are engaged in nursing education in each of the following disciplines, general, sick children's, psychiatric, mental handicap and public health, respectively, elected by nurses;

(c) five nurses resident in the State who are engaged in nursing management in each of the following disciplines, general, sick children's, psychiatric, mental handicap and public health, respectively, elected by nurses;

(d) three midwives resident in the State, one of whom is engaged in midwifery education, one of whom is engaged in midwifery management and one of whom is engaged in clinical practice, elected by midwives;

(e) three persons appointed by the Minister for Health and Children (the Minister), representative of the interests of the general public, who are not nurses or former nurses; and

(f) not more than four persons (other than candidates unsuccessful in elections to the Board) nominated by the Board at its discretion and appointed by the Minister, representative of any areas of the health services, or of nursing education, or of a category of nursing not elected to the Board. (4.21)

- The Commission recommends that the 1985 Act be amended to provide that the term of office for members of the Board be of six years duration with half the number going out of office every three years. (4.22)

- The Commission recommends that the Board consider the more active use of section 13 of the 1985 Act (relating to the establishment of committees) to broaden even further the range of expertise available to it in considering issues of concern to the profession. (4.26)

- The Commission recommends that the 1985 Act be amended to provide for revised fitness to practise procedures. The revised framework provides for the setting up of three ad hoc sub-committees drawn from the membership of the Fitness to Practise Committee. A person cannot be a member of more than one sub-committee dealing with the same complaint(s) under the revised fitness to practise procedures. (4.32)

- The Commission recommends that there should be an ad hoc preliminary screening sub-committee, composed of three members of the Fitness to Practise Committee. (4.33)

- If a complaint relates to a health issue, the Commission recommends that there should be an ad hoc health sub-committee, composed of five members of the Fitness to Practise Committee (one of whom must be a representative of the public interest) to investigate the issue. (4.34)

- If a complaint relates to a misconduct issue, the Commission recommends that there should be an ad hoc professional conduct sub-committee, composed of five members of the Fitness to Practise Committee (one of whom must be a representative of the public interest and one of whom must be of the same discipline as the nurse) to investigate the issue. (4.35)

- The Commission acknowledges the request from midwives for recognition of their distinct identity and recommends that the title of the amending legislation should be the Nurses and Midwives Act. (4.44)

- The Commission recommends the 1985 Act be amended to provide for the restoration of a separate statutory midwives committee consisting of eight members. It is recommended that such a committee consist of the three elected midwife members of the Board and five registered midwives appointed by the Board. In light of the increasing demand for domiciliary midwifery services, it is recommended that one of the five registered midwives appointed by the Board should be a midwife currently engaged in providing domiciliary midwifery services. This committee should have power to draft the scope of practice for midwives subject to approval of the Board. In the case of an allegation of professional misconduct against a midwife, four of the midwives committee plus one member of the Fitness to Practise Committee, representative of the interests of the general public, should be constituted by the Chair of the Fitness to Practise Committee as a professional conduct sub-committee reporting back to the Board with recommendations. At least one of the midwives on the professional conduct sub-committee should be an elected member of the Board. Health cases can be heard by a health sub-committee appointed in the normal way by the Chair of the Fitness to Practise Committee. (4.45)

- The Commission recommends that the 1985 Act be amended to entitle the Board to require any nurse or midwife to satisfy it as to her or his relevant competencies, failing which the Board could require an up-date on skills and knowledge, as a condition of retention of name on the register, provided the purpose would be for the protection of the public even in the absence of any complaint. Rules for the exercise of this power, which are fair and equitable, would have to be drawn up by the Board and monitored to ensure that the concerns expressed about its exercise would not be realised. (4.51)

- The Commission recommends that section 30 of the 1985 Act (which deals with regulation of a profession ancillary to nursing by the Board) be deleted. The Commission also recommends that the Minister establish a working party comprised of representatives of the Department of Health and Children, the Health Service Employers Agency, nursing and other appropriate organisations to establish standard criteria in relation to the entry requirements, education qualifications and training for care assistants across the health service. (4.55)

Main Recommendations on Preparation for the Profession

- The Commission recommends that the Minister facilitate the transition of pre-registration nursing education into third-level institutes at degree level. (5.19)

- The Commission recommends that the future framework for the pre-registration education of nurses be based on a four year degree programme in each of the disciplines of general, psychiatric and mental handicap nursing, approved by the Board, which will encompass clinical placements, including twelve months continuous clinical placement as a paid employee of the health service. (5.22)

- The Commission recommends that a forum be established by the Minister involving the third-level institutes, schools of nursing, health service providers and the Board. The objective of the forum should be to agree a strategy for the implementation of degree level pre-registration education and it should be funded by the State. The Minister, following consultation with the Minister for Education, Science and Technology, should appoint an independent chair of the forum. In addition the Commission recommends that the forum report within two years of its establishment. (5.26)

- The Commission recommends that all third-level institutes and disciplines of nursing should commence the pre-registration degree programme on a specified date. The Commission recommends that the start of the academic year in 2002 be specified as the commencement date of the degree programme. (5.30)

- The Commission recommends that the Central Applications Office (CAO) administer the application system for pre-registration nursing education. (5.34)

- The Commission recommends that the administration of the pre-registration nursing application system for the current diploma programmes be transferred to the CAO, in advance of the move to a third-level institute-based degree qualification. (5.35)

- The Commission recommends that admission to nursing be on the basis of the attainment of a specified Leaving Certificate standard plus an interview. (5.36)

- The Commission recommends that the Board have the responsibility of overseeing the interview process in the selection of candidates for the degree programme and keep the systems used in the selection of students for nursing under constant review to ensure the continuing use of best practice. The cost of administering the selection process should be met by the State. (5.41)

- The Commission recommends that the student nursing grant and any student benefits should be the same as those available to other third-level students and be means tested. (5.43)

- The Commission recommends that the student is paid a salary during the twelve months continuous clinical placement at the level of eighty percent of the first year staff nurse's salary. This is the current level of payment for third year apprenticeship students. The twelve months continuous clinical placement for which a student is paid should also be subsequently reckonable for pension purposes. Following graduation, the Commission recommends that a nurse, who has completed the twelve months continuous clinical placement, should start employment at the second increment point on the staff nurse salary scale. (5.44)

- The Commission recommends a bursary/sponsorship system be put in place by the Department of Health and Children to promote applications to all disciplines by mature students. (5.46)

- The Commission recommends that the Board and the Department of Health and Children examine mechanisms of promoting the profession as a career option among school leavers. (5.47)

- The Commission recommends that the Board examine mechanisms of increasing the number of male candidates applying to enter the profession. (5.48)

- The Commission recommends that health service employers consult with each nurse tutor currently involved in pre-registration nursing education in relation to her or his desired future career pathway. The purpose of the consultation is to establish whether the tutor wishes to move into third-level education or pursue other avenues in continuing education within the health service or other career options in management or clinical practice. The Commission recommends that health service providers support nurse tutors in upgrading their educational or other qualifications to facilitate their transition to their desired career pathway. (5.57)

- The Commission recommends, in order to facilitate the transition of as many nurse tutors as possible to the third-level sector, that those nurse tutors who may not have been successful in competing for academic posts within third-level institutes or who do not meet the academic and other requirements for appointment as a lecturer within the academic career structure of a third-level institute be appointed as "nurse lecturers" on a personal basis in a similar manner to that developed in Northern Ireland. (5.58)

- The Commission recommends that following the transition of pre-registration nursing education to a third-level degree programme, future nurse educators be appointed within the academic career structure of a third-level institute. (5.59)

- The Commission recommends that the schools of nursing become centres of nursing education providing a range of educational and training services to nurses in the health services. (5.61)

Main Recommendations on Professional Development

- The Commission recommends the Minister establish an independent statutory agency with responsibility for post-registration professional development of nursing and midwifery. The Commission recommends the independent statutory agency be called the National Council for the Professional Development of Nursing and Midwifery (the National Council). (6.12)

- The Commission recommends the National Council be given the following functions:

To:

- monitor the on-going development of nursing and midwifery specialities, taking into account, changes in practice and service need;

- establish guidelines for the creation of specialist nursing and midwifery posts by health service providers;

- determine the appropriate level of qualification and experience for entry into specialist nursing and midwifery practice (interim and long-term requirements);

- accredit specialist nursing and midwifery courses (including those provided independently by universities and colleges) for the purpose of appointment as a clinical nurse or midwife specialist or advanced nurse or midwife practitioner, taking account of: standards of professional practice and conduct set by the Board; geographic spread and access by nurses and midwives; and, in particular, service need;

- support additional developments in continuing nurse education by health boards and voluntary organisations;

- assist health service providers by setting guidelines for the selection of nurses and midwives who might apply for financial support in seeking opportunities to pursue further education;

- accredit post-registration courses (other than those courses leading to registration as a midwife, public health nurse, sick children's nurse or nurse tutor) for the purpose of recording on the register maintained by the Board;

- liaise with bodies in other jurisdictions in relation to the professional development of nursing and midwifery; and

- publish an annual report on its activities including the disbursement of monies by the Council. (6.14)

- The Commission recommends that the National Council be funded through the Department of Health and Children. (6.17)

- The Commission recommends that:

  - the National Council have a board of twenty members appointed by the Minister for a five year period;

  - members be limited to serving two consecutive terms on the National Council; of the first National Council appointed by the Minister, half of the membership be limited to serving one term of office;

  - on the first National Council appointed by the Minister, members limited to serving one term be selected by lottery on appointment;

  - the Chair be appointed by the Minister and that subsequent Chairs be elected by the members of the Board; and

  - the Chair have a five year term of office. (6.18)

- The Commission recommends that the Minister provide for the following membership of the National Council:

  - seven registered nurses, one from each of the following areas: general nursing, mental handicap nursing, psychiatric nursing, public health nursing, sick children's nursing, care of the elderly and a nurse tutor. The nurses appointed by the Minister from the various disciplines must be nurses of high professional standing with experience of advanced practice;

  - a registered midwife of high professional standing with experience of advanced practice;

  - two members of An Bord Altranais nominated by the Board;

  - one member following consultation with the Office for Health Management;

  - one senior nurse manager following consultation with the appropriate professional bodies;

  - two members following consultation with the Health Service Employers Agency;

  - two officers of the Department of Health and Children, one of whom shall be the Chief Nursing Officer at the Department;

- one medical practitioner following consultation with the Royal College of Surgeons, the Royal College of Physicians, the Irish College of General Practitioners and the Royal College of Psychiatrists in Ireland; and

- three nurses or midwives following consultation with third-level institutes, one of whom shall be the Head of a Department of Nursing in a NUI University, one shall be the Head of a Department of Nursing in a non-NUI University and one shall be the Head of a Department of Nursing in an Institute of Technology or a Regional Technical College. (6.19)

- The Commission recommends that the Minister provide that the contract of employment of every nurse and midwife in the public service, should entitle them to release, by an employer, for a minimum of two days paid study leave each year for continuing professional education. (6.23)

- The Commission recommends that the Minister provide for a three step clinical career path in nursing and midwifery. The Commission recommends the following clinical career pathway:

  - registered nurse/midwife;

  - clinical nurse or midwife specialist (CNS); and

  - advanced nurse or midwife practitioner (ANP). (6.26)

- The Commission recommends that for progression along the clinical career ladder, nurses and midwives must meet the practice and education guidelines set by the National Council. (6.27)

- The Commission recommends that to use either the title of "clinical nurse or midwife specialist" or "advanced nurse or midwife practitioner", a nurse or midwife must be appointed to a particular post. The recognition of CNS and ANP status must be matched with specified posts within the health services. (6.29)

- The Commission recommends that the Minister provide for a grade of clinical nurse or midwife specialist equivalent to ward sister level. The Commission recommends that the Minister also provide for a grade of advanced nurse or midwife practitioner equivalent to middle nursing and midwifery management level. The terms and conditions of employment should be determined through the normal channels. (6.30)

- The Commission recommends that programmes intending to prepare nurses and midwives for the role of CNS or ANP should have a large component of clinical practice (competency being assessed during the programme) and the programme should be accredited by the National Council. (6.50)

- The Commission recommends that when negotiating the move of post-registration programmes to third-level institutes, health service employers undertake a detailed consultation with the nurse educators currently involved in post-registration education programmes. Each nurse educator should be consulted in relation to her or his desired future career pathway whether she or he wishes to move into the third-level sector, pursue other avenues in professional development within the health service or other career options in management or clinical practice. The Commission recommends that health service providers support post-registration nurse educators in upgrading their education or other qualifications to facilitate their transition to their desired career pathway. (6.52)

- The Commission recommends that clinical nurse or midwife specialists undertake a relevant specialist post-registration university/college diploma and have extensive experience in the particular field of nursing or midwifery. (6.53)

- The Commission recommends that advanced nurse or midwife practitioners, who will be expected to conduct research into clinical nursing or midwifery issues, be prepared to masters degree level. (6.53)

- The Commission recommends that nurses and midwives with substantial specialist experience should be given accreditation for prior education and experience when seeking entry to specialist educational programmes. (6.55)

- The Commission recommends that in the initial filling of posts, where the recognition and establishment of a post or posts have been identified, those nurses and midwives practising at a specialist level, who satisfy the criteria established by the National Council (credit being given for prior education and experience) and are currently carrying out the duties of the approved post, should be appointed as clinical nurse or midwife specialists. (6.60)

- The Commission recommends that all concerned afford top priority to the creation of CNS and ANP posts. (6.61)

- The Commission recommends that the question of additional recognition of long service for staff nurses be examined through the established structures. (6.64)

- The Commission recommends that outstanding claims for allowances should be referred to the Labour Court for argument and determination as a matter of urgency. (6.66)

- The Commission recommends that the Minister provide for nursing and midwifery research to be funded through the Health Research Board (HRB). The Commission recommends that the Minister make funding available to the HRB specifically for nursing and midwifery research. (6.72)

- The Commission recommends that a comprehensive database of Irish nursing and midwifery research, funded by the State, be established. (6.74)

- The Commission recommends that the Minister appoint a registered nurse or midwife with experience in research to the board of the HRB. (6.75)

Main Recommendations on the Role of Nurses and Midwives in the Management of Services

- The Commission recommends that all health service providers put in place mechanisms for ensuring an effective internal communications system with nurses and midwives. Such systems should be audited on an on-going basis to ensure their continuing effectiveness in conveying and receiving information. (7.12)

- The Commission recommends that health service providers introduce systems to facilitate the development of personal career planning amongst nurses and midwives. (7.14)

- The Commission recommends the development of the post of Chief Nursing Officer at the Department of Health and Children. The post should be filled on a fixed-term contract basis. Given the crucial role of the post, the Commission recommends that the Chief Nursing Officer be supported by the recruitment of nurses and midwives from the health services. (7.16)

- The Commission recommends the establishment of a Nursing and Midwifery Planning and Development Unit in each health board. The Commission recommends the Nursing and Midwifery Planning and Development Unit have the following general functions:

- strategic planning and quality assurance of nursing and midwifery services in a health board area;

- co-ordinating the delivery of nursing and midwifery services and improving co-operation between health board and voluntary bodies in the delivery of nursing and midwifery services;

- working in partnership with the Chief Nursing Officer in the Department of Health and Children in planning and policy development on nursing and midwifery issues;

- overseeing the detailed provision of continuing nursing and midwifery education within a health board area;

- liaising with centres of nursing education within health service providers;

- developing, monitoring and reviewing the co-ordination and development of multi-disciplinary nursing services within a community care area;

- identifying inter-nursing disciplinary and inter-agency training needs and promoting the development of an inter-nursing disciplinary and inter-agency training strategy;

- reviewing significant issues in relation to inter-nursing disciplinary and inter-agency co-operation arising from the handling of selected cases; and

- assisting in improving internal communications with nurses and midwives in a health board area. (7.17)

- The Commission recommends that the Nursing and Midwifery Planning and Development Unit at health board level be headed by a senior nurse on a fixed-term contract - the Director of the Nursing and Midwifery Planning and Development Unit - who would report to the Chief Executive Officer of a health board. The post of Director of the Nursing and Midwifery Planning and Development Unit should be filled by interview following an open competition. (7.18)

- The Commission recommends that the nursing and midwifery staff of the Nursing and Midwifery Planning and Development Units be recruited from nursing and midwifery staff within a health board area for periods of up to two years. (7.18)

- The Commission recommends that the responsibilities of senior nursing and midwifery management should include:

- providing strategic and clinical leadership and direction for nursing and midwifery and related services which results in the delivery of effective, efficient, quality assured and patient centred nursing and midwifery care;

- developing a shared sense of commitment and participation amongst staff in the management of change, the development of nursing and midwifery services and in responding to the changing health needs of patients;

- developing the concept of care planning in collaboration with other professionals;

- participating in the overall financial planning of the health service provided including the assessment of priorities in pay and non-pay expenditure;

- ensuring that the appropriate in-service education programmes and on-going learning needs are met for all assigned staff; and

· ensuring that modern standards of clinical nursing and midwifery care are in operation and that regular monitoring of nursing and midwifery care is undertaken through audit. (7.20)

● The Commission recommends that in future all matrons in large acute hospitals and chief nursing officers in the psychiatric services should be entitled Directors of Nursing. (7.22)

● In order to discharge their general management functions more effectively, the Commission recommends that matrons of smaller hospitals should be given more explicit input into the determination of the budget and greater control and responsibility over its utilisation. (7.23)

● The Commission recommends that consideration should be given to the appointment of nurse or midwife managers as clinical directors, where appropriate. (7.27)

● The Commission recommends that middle nursing and midwifery management should:

  · have a defined management role and not merely retain a "gatekeeping" administrative function;

  · have defined management responsibility with explicit delegation of authority from directors of nursing and chief nursing officers;

  · have definite functional roles either in managing units of care or in the management of functional responsibilities such as in bed management and practice development co-ordination; and

  · have the authority to manage their area of responsibility without constant reference to more senior management. However, as in all management, there should be effective communication with front-line and senior management. (7.29)

● The Commission recommends that clerical and information technology support be made available to first line nursing and midwifery managers to support them in their managerial function, where appropriate. (7.36)

● The Commission recommends investment in the management information and support systems used by health service providers, to allow for greater devolution of budgetary responsibility which would result in significant improvements in the effective and efficient utilisation of resources. (7.38)

● The Commission recommends that training programmes should be organised in partnership between health boards, voluntary agencies and the Office for Health Management to develop and support existing first line nursing and midwifery managers to enable them to take on additional management and budgetary responsibilities. (7.40)

● The Commission recommends the development of first line nursing and midwifery management to fulfil the following functions:

  · professional/clinical leadership;

  · staffing and staff development;

  · resource management; and

  · facilitating communication. (7.41)

● The Commission recommends that first line nursing and midwifery managers should have management training before taking up a post and be required and supported in continuing to develop management skills. The development of management skills should operate in tandem with maintaining clinical credibility by being aware of changes in clinical practice. (7.41)

- The Commission recommends that there should be three grades of first line nursing and midwifery management in the health service, the title used to be "Clinical Nurse Manager" or "Clinical Midwife Manager". The three grades would be:

  - Clinical Nurse Manager 1 or Clinical Midwife Manager 1 (reporting to a Clinical Nurse or Midwife Manager 2);

  - Clinical Nurse Manager 2 or Clinical Midwife Manager 2 (in charge of a ward or unit of care); and

  - Clinical Nurse Manager 3 or Clinical Midwife Manager 3 (in charge of a department).

The conditions of employment of these posts should be determined in the appropriate fora. (7.45)

- The Commission recommends that differentials and incremental annual leave in promotional grades be looked at as a matter of urgency, before the end of December 1998, through the established structures. To this examination should be added the effect of the enhanced role for ward sisters and higher grades recommended by the Commission. (7.50)

- The Commission recommends that health service providers encourage nurses and midwives to seek opportunities in general management and that nurses and midwives consider pursuing careers in general health service management. (7.51)

- The Commission recommends that the Office for Health Management carry out a survey into the competencies required for nursing and midwifery management positions. (7.52)

- The Commission recommends that vacant management posts, where nurses and midwives are "acting-up", should be filled as soon as possible. (7.54)

- The Commission recommends that, where appropriate, nursing and midwifery management development programmes should be run in conjunction with management programmes for other professional groups and general managers. (7.57)

- The Commission recommends that the Health Service Employers Agency and nursing unions develop an agreed framework for the provision of permanent part-time contracts of employment for nurses and midwives. (7.62)

- The Commission recommends that the Health Service Employers Agency and nursing unions examine the equity of current arrangements for nurses and midwives seeking to move from one health board to another or from one hospital to another within a health board. (7.62)

- The Commission recommends that health service providers, nursing and midwifery management and nursing organisations examine opportunities for the increased use of care assistants and other non-nursing personnel in the performance of non-nursing tasks. (7.63)

- The Commission recommends that the Department of Health and Children, health service providers and nursing organisations examine the development of appropriate systems to determine nursing staffing levels. (7.63)

- The Commission recommends that vacant permanent posts should be filled without delay. A framework should be put in place, following discussions between the Health Service Employers Agency and nursing unions, to ensure the problem (the number of long-term temporary nurses in the health service) does not recur. (7.66)

- The Commission recommends the on-going development of occupational health programmes where they are currently provided and their introduction in areas of the health service where they are not currently available. (7.70)

- The Commission recommends that there should be long-term financial commitment to developing communication, management information and support systems to allow for greater devolution of budgets and staff development programmes. These programmes need to be underpinned by the allocation of adequate resources and a commitment to on-going funding. (7.78)

Main Recommendations on Nursing in the Community

- The Commission recommends that the Nursing and Midwifery Planning and Development Unit in each health board should develop strategies to improve communication and integration between nursing services in community care areas. (8.18)

- The Commission recommends that the Department of Health and Children issue a revised strategy statement on the role of public health nursing. The report *Public Health Nursing: A Review* (1997) should inform the deliberations on a revised strategy statement. (8.24)

- The Commission recommends the continuation of the present area-based model of public health nursing. However, the public health nurse (PHN) should be allowed focus to a greater extent on a health promotion and disease prevention role in the community. The Commission recommends that PHNs should receive greater support in their role through the provision of new technology and, where appropriate, clerical support. (8.27)

- The Commission recommends that, in light of the range of services offered by public health nurses and the ongoing development of nursing and midwifery services in the community, registration as a midwife should no longer be a mandatory requirement for entry to the higher diploma in public health nursing or registration as a public health nurse. An alternative education programme relating more closely to the core generic maternal and child care service requirements of public health nursing should replace the mandatory midwifery requirement. The Commission recommends that the Board establish a working party composed of PHNs, health service providers and nurse educators to determine the content and duration of a course in maternal and child health, as an alternative to the mandatory midwifery qualification. (8.30)

- The Commission recommends that the future role of the superintendent public health nurse should be concentrated on issues such as:

  - providing strategic and clinical leadership and direction for nursing and related services which results in the delivery of effective, efficient, quality assured and patient centred nursing care;

  - developing a shared sense of commitment and participation amongst staff in the management of change, the development of nursing services and in responding to the changing health needs of patients;

  - developing the concept of care planning in collaboration with other professionals;

  - participating in the overall financial planning of the health service provided including the assessment of priorities in pay and non-pay expenditure;

  - ensuring that appropriate in-service education programmes and on-going learning needs are met for all assigned staff; and

  - ensuring that modern standards of clinical nursing care are in operation and that regular monitoring of nursing care is undertaken through audit. (8.32)

- The Commission recommends that the title of Superintendent Public Health Nurse be changed to Director of Public Health Nursing and that the job description reflect the changing role. (8.33)

- The Commission recommends that senior public health nurses should:

  - have a defined management role and not merely retain a "gatekeeping" administrative function;

  - have defined management responsibility with explicit delegation of authority;

  - have definite functional roles in managing areas for the delivery of public health nursing services; and

  - have the authority to manage their area of responsibility without constant reference to more senior management, but as in all management, there should be effective communication with public health nurses and senior management. (8.35)

- The Commission recommends that the title of Senior Public Health Nurse be changed to Assistant Director of Public Health Nursing. (8.36)

- The Commission recommends that where registered general nurses are employed in the community it should be in a permanent capacity in line with service need. Such nurses should be employed in support of the public health nursing service as part of the community nursing team. Flexible permanent part-time employment opportunities could be provided to registered general nurses working in the community which would more effectively align service needs with the personal circumstances of such nurses. (8.38)

- The Commission recommends that health service providers and the National Council examine the development of clinical nurse specialisms with consequential posts which would enhance the delivery of mental handicap nursing services in the community. (8.43)

- The Commission recommends that an enhanced community psychiatric nursing service should provide for the development of clinical nurse specialists and advanced practitioners within the community in each catchment area throughout the country, according to service need. (8.52)

- The Commission recommends that the Nursing and Midwifery Planning and Development Unit, in planning the continuing professional development needs of nurses within a health board area, should also assist practice nurses in their professional development. (8.53)

- The Commission recommends that a practice nurse be attached on a sessional basis to the General Practice Unit within the health board to assist in identifying and supporting the development needs of practice nurses. (8.53)

Main Recommendations in Relation to Nursing in Care of the Elderly

- The Commission recommends that the Department of Health and Children examine, as a matter of urgency, conditions and staffing levels in care of the elderly services. (9.4)

- The Commission recommends that the Department of Health and Children review services for the elderly in each health board at the earliest opportunity. (9.4)

- The Commission recommends that centres of nursing education, in conjunction with third-level institutes, develop nurse education programmes to meet the needs of nurses working in care of the elderly. (9.5)

Main Recommendations in Relation to Certain Issues Concerning Mental Handicap Nursing, Midwifery and Sick Children's Nursing

- The Commission considers that there is a need to promote the distinct identity and unique working environment of mental handicap nursing and recommends that the Board develop a strategy, in consultation with nurse educators, mental handicap nurses and service providers, to promote mental handicap nursing as a career. (10.5)

- The Commission recommends that the Board review the current midwifery education programme as a matter of urgency. The review should, in particular, examine the length of the programme and the level of theoretical instruction provided to student midwives and compare such theoretical instruction with that required under a third-level post graduate higher diploma programme. (10.12)

- The Commission recommends that a direct entry midwifery course be piloted by the Board in a maternity hospital. Such a programme should initially be provided at diploma level but should move to a degree programme in 2002. (10.12)

- The Commission recommends that the statutory midwives committee within the Board, proposed in the revised regulatory framework, develop a scope of practice framework covering the activities of independent midwives in the community. Such a scope of practice should cover the professional requirements of a midwife practising in the community and address issues in relation to their on-going practice and clinical audit. (10.15)

- The Commission recommends that the qualification of sick children's nursing remain a post-registration qualification. However, prior to the transition of direct entry nursing disciplines to a degree programme, directors of nursing from the paediatric hospitals, sick children's nurse educators and the Board, should review the content, duration and academic award of the sick children's nursing course, in light of the proposed degree course curricula. (10.20)

- The Commission recommends that the title Sick Children's Nurse be changed to Child Health Nurse. (10.21)

Other Recommendations

- The Commission recommends that all health service employers develop formal and informal procedures to deal with bullying in the workplace. (11.11)

Main Recommendations on Implementation of the Report

- The Commission recommends the establishment of a monitoring committee under the aegis of the Department of Health and Children comprising representatives of the Department, the Board, the four nursing unions and service providers to monitor the progress of the implementation of the recommendations. The Commission recommends that progress reports on the implementation of the recommendations be prepared annually for circulation among the profession. (12.2)

- The Commission recommends a timetable in relation to certain key institutional and structural reforms (including the following):

  - the legislation amending the Nurses Act 1985 should be introduced before the Houses of the Oireachtas by early 1999;

- the forum composed of representatives of the third-level institutes, schools of nursing, health service providers and the Board should be established at the earliest possible date;

- the degree programme should commence at the start of the academic year in 2002;

- the National Council for the Professional Development of Nursing and Midwifery should be established at the earliest possible date;

- the Nursing and Midwifery Planning and Development Units in each health board should be put in place at the earliest possible date. (12.3)

Introduction

Chapter

1

Introduction

Terms of Reference and Membership of Commission

1.1 The Commission on Nursing was established by the Minister for Health, Mr. Michael Noonan T.D., on 21 March 1997 following a recommendation from the Labour Court (Recommendation No. LCR15450). During its deliberations on a series of issues in dispute between health service employers and the Nursing Alliance, the Labour Court recognised that there had been extensive changes in the requirements placed on nurses, both in training and in the delivery of services. The Labour Court recommended that both the Nursing Alliance and the health service employers be involved in agreeing the terms of reference which would be wide ranging and include addressing such items as structural and work changes, segmentation of the grade, training and education requirements, promotional opportunities and related difficulties and a general assessment of the evolving role of nurses.

1.2 The terms of reference of the Commission were agreed as follows:

The Commission will examine and report on the role of nurses in the health service including:

- *the evolving role of nurses, reflecting their professional development and their role in the overall management of services;*

- *promotional opportunities and related difficulties;*

- *structural and work changes appropriate for the effective and efficient discharge of that role;*

- *the requirements placed on nurses, both in training and the delivery of services;*

- *segmentation of the grade; and*

- *training and education requirements.*

In its recommendations it should seek to provide a secure basis for the further professional development of nursing in the context of anticipated changes in health services, their organisation and delivery.

1.3 In light of discussions during the consultative process undertaken by the Commission and following the agreement of the Board, the Commission sought an extension of its terms of reference to include:

the role and function of An Bord Altranais generally, including, inter alia, education and professional development, regulation and protection of the citizen.

The Minister for Health and Children, Mr. Brian Cowen T.D., agreed to the above on 12 September, 1997.

1.4 The Minister for Health, Mr. Michael Noonan T.D., appointed the following persons to be members of the Commission:

Chair: Ms. Justice Mella Carroll

Members: Dr. Ruth Barrington, Assistant Secretary, Department of Health and Children

              Mr. Leslie Buckley, Management Consultant

              Ms. Kay Collins, Staff Nurse, University College Hospital, Galway

Mr. Denis Doherty, Chief Executive Officer, Midland Health Board

Ms. Antoinette Doocey, Public Health Nurse, North-Eastern Health Board

Ms. Sandra Guilfoyle, Personnel Consultant

Mr. Philip Halpin, Chief Operating Officer, National Irish Bank

Ms. Eilish Hardiman, Ward Sister, St. James's Hospital

Mr. Des Kavanagh, General Secretary, Psychiatric Nurses Association

Mr. P.J. Madden, General Secretary, Irish Nurses Organisation

Dr. Geraldine McCarthy-Haslam, Head of Department of Nursing Studies, National University of Ireland, Cork

Dr. David McCutcheon, Chief Executive Officer, The Adelaide and Meath Hospitals, Dublin, incorporating The National Children's Hospital

Mr. Leo O'Donnell, Chartered Accountant

Ms. Peta Taaffe, Chief Nursing Officer, Department of Health and Children

1.5 Dr. David McCutcheon resigned from the Commission on 23 May 1997 because of an increased workload associated with revised plans for the opening of the hospital in Tallaght. It is with regret that the Commission noted Dr. McCutcheon's resignation.

1.6 Mr. Philip Halpin resigned from the Commission on 17 June 1998 due to increased work commitments. It is with regret that the Commission noted Mr. Halpin's resignation and wishes to record its appreciation for his valuable input to the Commission.

1.7 The members of the secretariat to the Commission were as follows:

Mr. Dermot McCarthy, Secretary (seconded from the Department of Health and Children).

Ms. Geraldine Graham, Deputy Secretary (seconded from the Midland Health Board).

Ms. Maureen Flynn, Researcher (seconded from St. Vincent's Hospital, Elm Park).

Ms. Lynda Gavin, Clerical Officer (seconded from the Eastern Health Board).

Mr. Pat Preston, Usher to Ms. Justice Mella Carroll, High Court.

1.8 The Commission would like to record its gratitude and indebtedness to all members of the secretariat, each of whom contributed in a special way to the completion of the final work of the Commission.

Thanks are due to:

● Dermot for his dedication and unstinting hard work and his success in encapsulating in elegant prose the wide ranging discussions of the Commission;

● Geraldine whose abilities and general initiative (showing immense future potential) made her the ideal deputy;

● Maureen who brought her considerable skills to bear in producing impeccable research and who kept the Commission up-to-date in relevant information;

- Lynda who among her all round skills, was the "voice" of the Commission to the outside world and who speedily and efficiently produced drafts and copies of documents necessary for the work of the Commission; and

- Pat who successfully took on a wide variety of jobs as they presented, who looked after the complexities of moving the Commission around the country and who ensured the members were well looked after at all times

and to all of them collectively for creating the happy atmosphere which existed at 21 Fitzwilliam Square throughout the life of the Commission.

Consultative Process

1.9 Throughout its lifetime, the Commission consulted widely with nurses and midwives, and other interested parties through the following media:

- written submissions;

- consultative fora;

- meetings with individuals and groups;

- seminars following publication of the interim report; and

- meetings with stakeholders prior to the publication of the final report.

1.10 The Commission placed advertisements in national and provincial newspapers inviting written submissions from interested parties. Almost 800 submissions were received and these are listed in appendix one. The submissions, from a range of individuals, groups and national bodies also provided an essential resource to the Commission in the identification of issues for consideration within its terms of reference and were used by the Commission in its deliberations prior to the publication of the final report.

1.11 At the outset, a series of consultative fora was organised with substantial assistance from health boards. Three sessions per day were held at thirteen venues throughout the country between 10th May and 14th June 1997 and approximately 3,000 people attended. While the vast majority of these were nurses from all disciplines, there was also a small number of other professionals in attendance, including doctors, pharmacists, career guidance teachers and occupational therapists. Participants were randomly assigned to a workshop, with each workshop choosing its own chair and rapporteur. In advance of each forum, questions were circulated for consideration to enable those attending to have a focused consultation in advance with colleagues who could not attend. The consultative fora proved very useful to the Commission in identifying a range of issues within its terms of reference.

1.12 The Commission also invited a number of persons to meet with it to discuss issues within its terms of reference. Valuable insights into particular areas of nursing and midwifery were gained through meeting with people who had varying perspectives on the development of nursing. A list of those invited to meet the Commission is at appendix two. The Commission would like to thank all who assisted it in its deliberations.

1.13 ## Interim Report

The Commission was requested to publish an interim report within six months of its establishment. The report, which reflected the initial phase of the work of the Commission, was published in October 1997 and concentrated on identifying the issues raised by the nursing profession and others during the consultative fora and in written submissions. The issues identified were complex and many were inter-related, while some reflected broader issues within the health and public service generally. The Commission considered these and other issues during the second stage of its work and addresses them in the context of its terms of reference in this, the final report.

Regional Seminars

1.14   Following the publication of the interim report, the Commission organised a series of seminars in November 1997, inviting individuals and representatives of groups who had forwarded written submissions and those who had attended meetings with the Commission. The focus of these seminars was to discuss in workshops the issues raised in the interim report and to ask those present to consider, whether in their view, the issues before the nursing profession had been correctly identified in the interim report and to propose possible solutions. It was decided to assign people to workshops according to discipline (as far as possible) to enable more focused discussion on the issues most pertinent to their particular area of work. Approximately 600 persons attended the seminars which were held on the following dates:

Monday, 10 November 1997 in the Silver Springs Hotel, Cork;

Wednesday, 12 November 1997 in the Grand Hotel, Malahide, Dublin; and

Friday, 14 November 1997 in the Hillgrove Hotel, Monaghan.

Meetings with Stakeholders

1.15   In the weeks prior to the publication of the final report, the Commission held meetings with a number of persons with an interest in nursing. The Commission also held a number of meetings with the Board. The persons invited to meet the Commission had previously made submissions or met the Commission during the consultative process and represented the broad spectrum of nursing and midwifery, and related interests. At the meetings, the Commission outlined proposals under consideration and sought the views of the stakeholders.

Visit to Australia

1.16   A visit, by five members of the Commission on Nursing, to Australia to meet with nursing and midwifery leaders and educators, was arranged in light of the reviews of international literature undertaken by the Commission. The literature reviews had identified that in Australia pre-registration nursing education had moved into the tertiary education sector and nursing graduates were awarded a degree-level qualification. In addition, the literature identified that a clinical career pathway had been developed in Australia with grades of clinical nurse specialist and clinical nurse consultant. These developments had taken place in the past ten years and whilst they had been identified in the literature, there was a paucity of material critically analysing these developments and their impact on nursing and midwifery and the health services in general. In meeting those directly involved in the management and education of nurses and midwives, it was hoped to obtain insights which would assist the Commission in its consideration of future education and career pathways for the profession.

1.17   The Commission met with nurse and midwife leaders and educators from throughout Australia and New Zealand. The openness and assistance offered to the Commission during the visit was much appreciated. Many nurse and midwife leaders travelled long distances to meet with the Commission and their insight into developments in Australia and New Zealand was of great assistance. The

Commission would particularly like to thank Ms. Suzanne Williams, Chief Nursing Officer, Health Department of Western Australia and Ms. Judith Meppem, Chief Nursing Officer, New South Wales Health Department for their help in organising the visit of the Commission to Australia.

1.18   The itinerary of the Commission during the visit to Australia was as follows:

Monday, 16 March 1998:

● Meeting with Chief Nursing Officers from the Australian States and New Zealand.

● Meeting joined by area/hospital Directors of Nursing in New South Wales.

Tuesday, 17 March 1998:

● Meeting with Australian Council of Deans of Nursing.

● Meeting with Nurses Registration Board of New South Wales.

Wednesday, 18 March 1998:

● Visit to Faculty of Nursing, the University of Newcastle, New South Wales.

● Visit to John Hunter Hospital, New South Wales.

Thursday, 19 March 1998:

● Meeting with Professor Christine Duffield, Faculty of Nursing, University of Technology, Sydney.

● Visit to the new Children's Hospital, Parramatta, Sydney.

Friday, 20 March 1998:

● Visit to Central Sydney Area Health Services:

    ‣ Queen Elizabeth II Centre;

    ‣ Royal Prince Alfred Hospital;

    ‣ Rozelle Hospital, Psychiatric Services;

    ‣ King George V, Maternity Services;

    ‣ Redfern, Community Health Centre.

Monday, 23 March 1998:

● Meeting with Royal College of Nursing, Canberra.

● Meeting with representatives of the Department of Health and Family Services and the Department of Employment, Education, Training and Youth Affairs.

A detailed list of those with whom the Commission met is at appendix three.

Meetings of the Commission

1.19   As well as the meetings described heretofore, the Commission met as a body on forty occasions throughout its lifetime.

1.20   As the issues emerged through the written submissions and consultative fora, the Commission decided to undertake some of its work by sub-committee. Initially two sub-committees were formed - one dealing with management issues and the second with professional development. Both sub-committees met on seven occasions prior to the interim report.

1.21   Following the extension of its terms of reference to include the role and function of the Board, the Commission decided to regroup into three sub-committees following the interim report:

● the management sub-committee, which met thirteen times;

● the education sub-committee, which met twelve times; and

● the regulation sub-committee, which met seven times.

1.22   The sub-committees produced discussion documents for consideration by the full Commission and these ultimately formed the basis of many chapters in this report.

Literature Reviews Undertaken by the Commission

1.23   In order to place nursing in its proper context both nationally and internationally, reviews of literature were commissioned as follows:

(i) *Changes in the Professional Role of Nurses in Ireland: 1980 - 1997* (Written by: Sarah Condell, Principal Nurse Tutor, The Adelaide and Meath Hospital, Dublin, incorporating the National Children's Hospital).

to identify changes in the professional role of nurses in Ireland; to identify the main social, demographic, legislative, educational and technological developments in Ireland which have impacted on the professional role of nurses in the last seventeen years.

(ii) *An Examination of the Changes in the Professional Role of the Nurse Outside Ireland* (Written by: Ellen B. Savage, Lecturer, Department of Nursing Studies, National University of Ireland, Cork).

to identify the changes, if any, that have taken place internationally in the professional role of nurses which would be of relevance to the professional development of nurses in Ireland. To examine, in particular, any changes that have recently taken place in the United Kingdom. To critically analyse changes which have taken place in other countries and suggest examples of good practice.

(iii) *Management in the Health Services: The Role of the Nurse* (Written by: Maureen Flynn, Anaesthetic Sister, Course Co-ordinator, St. Vincent's Hospital, Elm Park, Dublin).

to examine the role of nurses in the management of health services both in Ireland and internationally. In reviewing literature on international developments to concentrate on developments in the United Kingdom, Europe, North America and Australia/New Zealand, which are of relevance to the role of nurses in the management of the health services in Ireland.

(iv) *Developments in Pre-Registration Nursing Education - An International Perspective* (Written by: Mark Tyrrell, Lecturer, Department of Nursing Studies, National University of Ireland, Cork).

to conduct a review of the literature on current developments in nurse education in the United Kingdom, Australia, Canada and Europe (especially Denmark) paying particular attention to:

● Degree level preparation (generic or specialist);

● Selection;

● Relationship between third-level colleges and

- statutory bodies (e.g. curriculum and examinations) etc;

- schools of nursing/hospitals (re-clinical placements) etc;

- funding agencies;

- outcome evaluation.

● Process of merging/linking with third-level colleges.

If possible to give a general overview of nursing education in the United States of America.

(v) *Community Nursing - An International Perspective* (Written by: Patricia Leahy-Warren, Public Health Nurse, Southern Health Board).

to conduct a review of the literature on community nursing - service models, care delivery, management of, education for, financing etc. with particular reference to literature from the U.K., USA, Australia, Canada and Europe, especially Finland.

(vi) *Joint Appointments in Nursing* (Written by: Patricia Leahy-Warren and Mark Tyrrell).

to conduct a literature review on models for the appointment of nurse educators to joint positions with health service providers and third-level institutes.

1.24   The Commission wishes to acknowledge the dedication of these researchers in producing high calibre work. The literature reviews outlined above will be published separately to the report and have been edited by Dr. Geraldine McCarthy-Haslam, to whom the Commission extends its thanks.

1.25   The Commission wishes to thank Dr. Joe Robins, Social Historian and former Assistant Secretary in the Department of Health, for researching and writing chapter two on the evolution of the nursing profession in Ireland until the early 1980's, and the Central Statistics Office for their assistance in carrying out a survey of public satisfaction with nursing services.

1.26   The Commission wishes to record its appreciation to the following who were invited to submit discussion documents outlining their views on a framework for the future development of nursing in the community:

Jean Clarke, Co-ordinator Higher Diploma in Nursing Studies (Public Health Nursing), Department of Nursing Studies, National University of Ireland, Dublin;

Catherine McTiernan, Assistant Chief Nursing Officer, Mental Health Services, Eastern Health Board; and

Netta Williams, Practice Nurse, Department of General Practice, Royal College of Surgeons, Dublin.

1.27   The Commission also wishes to record its thanks to Leesha O'Driscoll and Milada Bacik, Law Researchers in the Judge's Library in the Four Courts, who undertook legal research on behalf of the Commission.

The Evolution of the Nursing Profession in Ireland until the early 1980's

Chapter 2

The Evolution of the Nursing Profession in Ireland until the Early 1980's

Formation Of The Profession

2.1   Three major influences shaped the development of nursing as a profession in Ireland - the religious orders of nursing sisters, scientific progress in the prevention and treatment of illness and disease and the life and writings of Florence Nightingale.

2.2   The lifting of the penal restrictions on the Catholic population in the early nineteenth century encouraged the founding of new Irish religious orders, notably the Sisters of Mercy and the Irish Sisters of Charity, who initiated new hospitals and other services for the sick poor. As well as managing these hospitals and services, the sisters also provided the nursing care. They were disciplined, highly dedicated women who advanced the hitherto low level of nursing care by their compassion and religious zeal. These orders promoted nursing the poor as a vocation and succeeded in attracting many young and well educated women from middle class families. St. Vincent's and the Mater Hospitals in Dublin, the Mater Infirmorum in Belfast and the Mercy Hospital in Cork came to be regarded in the second half of the nineteenth century as very caring institutions. This was in sharp contrast to the harsh attitudes and spartan standards which were a feature of the poor law workhouses established by local authorities in the 1830's and 1840's.

2.3   One of the most important developments in the nineteenth century for public health was the understanding that the transmission of disease was linked to sanitary conditions. Public health legislation, applied to Ireland as well as Britain, was promoting an increasingly cleaner, less hazardous, environment through the control of sewage, the introduction of clean water supplies and the reduction of insanitary conditions, especially in urban areas. During the 1860's, Louis Pasteur discovered germs and further scientific research led to the identification of the specific organisms giving rise to most of the main infectious diseases.

2.4   The concept of the hospital and care within the hospital were notably influenced by these advances. The sources and manner of transmission of infection impacted on the regimen of the hospital; the introduction of public sanitation and safe water supplies advanced the creation of better quality hospital accommodation; the development of antiseptics reduced the hazard of "hospital" diseases and of cross-infection. Adding further to the quality of hospital care was the discovery and introduction of anaesthesia, the beginning of painless surgery. As a result of these changes the late nineteenth century hospital had moved far beyond the relatively primitive institutions and notions of care of the earlier part of the century. New forms of care and therapy became possible. Hygiene became a paramount consideration. The knowledge and the skills, now accessible to the hospital, clearly demanded a body of trained and disciplined nurses to participate in their implementation. While, in the past, care in hospitals had been exclusively for the sick poor, since the better off could be looked after in their homes, now the higher quality of care and therapy becoming available could be provided only in a hospital setting.

2.5   It would be difficult to overstate the contribution of Florence Nightingale to the creation of a profession of nursing. When, during the 1850's, she was developing her ideas on this issue, she visited Dublin and saw the St. Vincent's services in operation. She had hoped to be admitted for training but the sisters were not prepared to admit lay trainees. Nightingale's efforts and ideas provided guidelines that moulded and enriched the new profession, not only in Britain and Ireland but throughout Western society. The original Nightingale school was opened at St. Thomas' hospital in London in 1860. Its programme was considerably influenced by the public health reforms of the period and by the recognition given to the importance of public and personal hygiene in the control of disease.

2.6   Florence Nightingale's main objective was to create a body of nurses capable of training others. The new nurses were expected, not to undertake private nursing but, to take posts in hospitals and other public caring institutions in order to establish a higher standard of nursing practice in them by passing on their training to their colleagues. It was in this way that her influence was felt in Irish hospitals. Those seeking admittance as probationers to the Nightingale School had to undergo stringent scrutiny and were required to come from "respectable" families, to have high moral standards and to be generally of unblemished character. Given attitudes to women in the Victorian era, it was critical to her strategy of developing the profession of nursing that its practitioners should be above reproach, both in their personal lives and on the wards. While the religious orders succeeded in promoting nursing as a vocation for sisters, Florence Nightingale's achievement was in promoting nursing as a profession for lay women.

The First Nursing Schools

2.7   Encouraged by the example of the Nightingale school in London and by the public health reforms and scientific discoveries of the period, most of the Irish voluntary hospitals had nurse training schemes in operation by the end of the century. The first training scheme in Dublin, influenced by the new criteria and techniques for nursing, was established by the Adelaide Hospital in 1858 with the guidance of an Englishwoman who had worked in the Crimea with Nightingale. Other training schemes followed. The Institute of Nursing, founded in 1866 by Frances Mary Trench, wife of the Protestant Archbishop of Dublin, became associated with Dr. Steevens' Hospital where practical training for probationers was provided. When this arrangement was ended the hospital took probationer nurses for some years from a training school established at Usher's Quay in 1881 by a Mrs. Brown from Merrion Square. These nurses became known as "Mrs. Brown's nurses", but Steevens' eventually decided to have its own nurse training in 1890. The Royal City of Dublin Hospital (Baggot Street) opened its own training scheme in 1884. In 1885, the Meath Hospital established the Dublin Red Cross Nursing Sisters' Home and Training School for Nurses in Harcourt Street. During the 1890's the Dublin Metropolitan School of Nursing was established largely due to the efforts of Margaret Huxley, Matron of Sir Patrick Dun's Hospital, where probationer nurses from Duns and other hospitals, including Mercer's, were trained. There had been some initial resistance to the introduction of trained nurses into the House Industry Hospitals (Richmond, Hardwicke, Whitworth) by the management board which was funded by government grant, but in 1892 the board reported that "intelligent and thoroughly reliable nurses" were being trained in the hospitals. In the early years of the new century the Victoria Hospital, Cork had a course of training for its nurses under way.

2.8   Prior to the 1890's the nursing duties of the religious owned hospitals were carried out by the nuns from their communities although lay personnel were employed as assistants. Up to this time there were no nurse training schemes within these institutions although the nuns received informal tuition and guidance within their own communities. As formal schemes of training associated with the lay operated hospitals continued to develop and expand, the Catholic Archbishop of Dublin took the initiative of asking the religious-controlled hospitals to establish schools for the training of young girls in the nursing profession. The Mater Hospital opened a school in 1891 and during the same year, the Charitable Infirmary (Jervis Street), also staffed by the Sisters of Mercy, opened a school. During 1892 St. Vincent's Hospital established a school in an adjacent premises and by 1909 was training religious from other orders as well as young lay girls.

2.9   Training was usually imbued with the distinctive culture of the individual hospital and consisted, in effect, of an apprenticeship where a large number of young trainees learned their skills from a small number of senior nurses while turning their hands to everything in the hospital wards. Young women entering the world of nursing found themselves in a strictly disciplined, regimented environment where good behaviour, obedience and dedication to their vocation were absolute requirements. Many of them were working in religious controlled hospitals where the regimen and restrictions imposed by their superiors bore comparison with that of a religious community. But, if the disciplines imposed by the nursing managements of the religious hospitals were strict, so too were those of the boards and matrons of the lay hospitals.

Sick Children's Nursing

2.10   Concern about the welfare of children was a notable feature of the strengthening philanthropy of the later nineteenth century. To some extent, this concern manifested itself in the establishment of children's hospitals. In Dublin, the first special hospitals of this sort were the National Children's Hospital, Harcourt Street (originally based on other sites) and The Children's Hospital, Temple Street. The introduction of these hospitals gave rise to the need for the special training of sick children's nurses. The earliest special training programme was established in 1893 at Temple Street.

Psychiatric Nursing

2.11   During the nineteenth century, a large number of psychiatric hospitals or asylums were built to provide accommodation for the mentally ill. The prevailing attitude in Victorian times was that the purpose of care in the asylums was confinement since there was little effective treatment for mental illness. The hospitals or asylums were staffed largely by attendants, with male staff looking after male patients and female staff caring for female patients. With few exceptions, the religious orders did not get involved in running psychiatric hospitals and psychiatry did not at this period experience the same degree of scientific progress as medicine and surgery. The absence of these two factors probably accounts for the later emergence of formal training for those caring for the mentally ill.

2.12   In the 1890's, the then medical superintendent of the Richmond Asylum (Grangegorman) insisted that attendants seeking promotion should pass an examination, but the Richmond was not typical and up to the end of the century there were few trained staff in the asylums. Most of the medical superintendents appeared indifferent to the need for formal training of the attendant staff. In general, this continued to be the situation up to the 1920's. The Royal Medico-Psychological Association provided courses for training and issued certificates but participation in the training depended largely on the encouragement given by the superintendents. Sometimes none was given. In any event, there was little inducement to attendants to undertake the examinations since for a considerable period the acquisition of a certificate meant an increase of only two pounds annually in their wages.

Midwifery

2.13   The evolution of midwifery was different to that of other branches of the profession. The process of childbirth had always been regarded as a natural event, unrelated to sickness: midwifery was seen as a special and exclusive skill related to that event. The home was accepted as the proper environment for birth and there was no great demand for the provision of institutional accommodation for that purpose. The small number of maternity hospitals, established in Ireland during the eighteenth and nineteenth centuries, were viewed by their founders and supporters as being exceptional measures to help mothers in the dire conditions prevailing in the overcrowded and squalid city tenements. The statistics of death for mothers and infants demonstrated ample evidence of the increased hazards of the city and the maternity hospitals provided alternative accommodation for those most at risk. While, as yet, there were no statutory controls on the practice of midwifery, courses of training were given in the hospitals, notably in the Rotunda

Hospital which had been offering instruction from the end of the eighteenth century for those wishing to acquire "not only a competent knowledge of the common practice of a midwife but of those accidents and extraordinary occurrences sometimes attendant on parturition".

2.14   In rural areas during the nineteenth century and the early decades of the present century almost all women underwent their confinements in their own home, no matter what their social class or their living conditions. During much of this period, if assistance was required, a call was made on the services of the local "handywoman", who had a long-established traditional role as the fount of all knowledge and skill as regards childbirth. Many of them had inherited certain skills passed down through their family line but their competence was variable. The first step towards the improvement of the midwifery services followed from the establishment of the dispensary system in 1851, when over seven hundred district doctors were appointed with responsibilities that included the care of maternity cases. The local boards of guardians who directed the dispensary services were encouraged by the central authorities to appoint midwives and despite considerable resistance by the guardians, largely on grounds of cost, there were 605 midwives in dispensary districts in 1905. But the midwives were poorly paid and mostly untrained and this continued to be the situation for a long time.

Public Health Nursing

2.15   While there was a certain amount of home visiting of the sick poor by the religious orders during the nineteenth century, the origins of district nursing derived, in the main, from the provisions for midwifery which accompanied the establishment of the dispensary doctor system. Towards the end of the century, a number of voluntary initiatives were taken which involved not only the provision of maternity care but the visiting of the sick in general. The main initiative undertaken was the establishment in 1890 of Queen Victoria's Jubilee Institute for Nurses. The Institute was funded with the contributions made to commemorate the golden jubilee of the queen's reign and its object was to provide a district nursing service in selected poorer districts largely in rural areas. Later in 1903, Lady Dudley, wife of the serving lord-lieutenant, founded a smaller but similar scheme intended for areas not already provided for, mainly in western and north-western parts of the country. The nurses appointed to both schemes were trained in general nursing and midwifery. The schemes were administered by the headquarters of the Institute in Dublin and the maintenance of the services were dependent to a considerable degree on local fund raising committees unassisted by support from public finance.

The Status of Irish Nursing in the Early Twentieth Century

2.16   By the early years of the twentieth century Irish nursing had been soundly established as a profession: a body of carefully chosen women, who were trained, disciplined and of unquestionable character. They were predominantly of middle-class origin. Apart from the Nightingale commendation that girls of good breeding should be chosen for the profession, the social attitudes of the period were an influence on the choice of nursing as a career. In the extremely class-conscious society of the times there was a degree of resistance among many middle-class and upper-class families to the notion of their daughters going out to work and earning a wage. Many occupations were seen as having unacceptable working-class connotations that breached the usually recognised dividing lines between the social classes, but following the reform of the profession, a career in nursing became acceptable. Voluntary charity work had become part of the usual social activity of young women of better off families during the latter part of the nineteenth century. Nursing was seen as a progression in that direction. It combined a caring activity with a career; with the further attraction that its training and experience could be a beneficial preparation for marriage. Remuneration was a secondary consideration.

2.17 The first professional nursing organisation, the Irish Matron's Association, was founded in 1904. The purpose of the Association was to enable matrons to discuss professional issues, to seek a uniform system of education and training and to monitor legislative proposals affecting the interests of the profession.

The First Phase of Regulation of the Profession

2.18 Midwifery was the first branch of the profession to be subject to regulation. Because of the activities of untrained midwives, the government provided in 1902 for the regulation of midwifery practice in Britain, including the phasing out of uncertified midwives, but the provisions were not extended to Ireland. Eventually, largely due to pressure from the Royal College of Physicians in Ireland, the government implemented measures for Ireland through the Midwives (Ireland) Act 1918. The new legislation forbade women, with effect from the beginning of 1919, to describe themselves as midwives unless qualified to do so. It also provided that, from the beginning of 1924, it would be an offence for a person, habitually and for gain, to attend a childbirth other than under the direction of a doctor, unless she was a certified midwife. A Central Midwives Board was established to oversee the operation of the new laws. However, it was well into the 1930's before the practice of midwifery by handywomen was finally eliminated. The Board remained as a separate authority, unrelated to the general body of nursing, until it was dissolved and its role integrated in that of An Bord Altranais (The Nursing Board) in 1951, but with provision for a special midwives committee.

2.19 In the early years of the twentieth century, there were strengthening demands in Britain and Ireland for the introduction of statutory controls to regulate and supervise the nursing profession in general. A parliamentary select committee, established in 1904, received representations from various interests that the registration of nurses was desirable. The parliamentary committee recommended the establishment of statutory machinery for the control and registration of nurses including the recognition of training schools and the conduct of examinations.

2.20 The years of the first world war postponed further action, but following the introduction of UK legislation, the Nurses' Registration (Ireland) Act 1919 established the General Nursing Council for Ireland. The new body, whose members were appointed by Government, was given responsibility for keeping registers of general nurses, nurses trained in psychiatric nursing and nurses trained in sick children's nursing. Training hospitals were subjected to recognition and the content of training and the conduct of examinations became subject to regulation. The regulation of general nursing remained separate from midwifery which continued to have its own supervisory system.

2.21 The legislation regulating nursing and midwifery emphasised supervision and control. It contrasted with that governing the medical and legal professions which permitted self regulation.

Conditions of Employment

2.22 For a considerable period, the pay of nurses compared poorly with that of other professions. There was the often unspoken attitude that because they were willing members of a dedicated vocation, with high marriage prospects and therefore the likelihood of short careers, they were unlikely to seek, or expect, anything better than a low level of pay. After a pay increase in 1925, nurses on the staffs of local authority hospitals still had only a salary of fifty pounds annually raising by increments to sixty-seven pounds. There were major adjustments in the years that followed but by 1944 the local authority nurses were still only on an annual scale of seventy-five pounds to ninety pounds. Voluntary hospitals, with less assured funding, often paid lower rates and most of them had no pension schemes for their staff. In 1945, the Hospitals Commission reported that two thirds of serving nurses were not then in pensionable positions.

2.23   Historically the nursing profession had always been reluctant to resort to industrial agitation to seek better pay and conditions excepting the militancy, including strikes, of the largely attendant staffs of mental hospitals in the decade that followed the founding in 1917 of the Irish Asylum Workers Union. The first move towards organising general nurses began with the founding of the Irish Nurses Union in 1919 as a branch of the Irish Women Workers Union. It was a daring move for the twenty Dublin nurses and midwives who came together to take the initiative at a time when their employers and many of their professional colleagues would have found incompatible the notion of trade union membership and the occupation of nursing. Later, the nurses' union severed its connection with the parent union and called itself The Irish Nurses Association: and still later, in 1949, it was renamed The Irish Nurses Organisation (INO). For a considerable period the Association (Organisation) distanced itself from the notion of taking on the full characteristics of a trade union because its members considered that they were precluded by their professional responsibility and ethical code from taking strike action. However, in 1942, it was granted registration as a trade union with limited powers of negotiation under the Trade Union Act 1941 and with that status continued to campaign strongly on behalf of nursing interests. This remained the situation until the Organisation was granted full registration as a trade union in 1988 and later affiliated to the Irish Congress of Trade Unions. While the INO remains the largest body representing nurses in Ireland there is substantial nurse membership in a number of other unions, notably, in SIPTU, IMPACT and the Psychiatric Nurses Association.

Development of Nursing and Midwifery in the Twentieth Century

2.24   Nursing has benefited from the gradual expansion and improvement of health and medical services that has taken place throughout this century. The development of a modern hospital system, beginning in the 1930's, created new opportunities for nurses and a growing demand for their services. It encouraged the growth of schools of nursing-based in hospitals throughout the country. Given the lack of employment opportunities for women over much of the period, there was no shortage of candidates for nursing.

2.25   The ending of the second world war in 1945 marked the beginning of a new era of social advance in most western countries. The concept of the welfare state emerged; there was a growing emphasis on equality and equity for all citizens: the State was seen as having the primary responsibility for safeguarding and promoting the welfare of the individual. As elsewhere, there was a rapidly increasing expansion of social services in Ireland, particularly in the health area, not just because of the acceptance of socialist philosophies but because of technological and scientific advances. The separate Department of Health was established in 1947 to deal with the growing provision of health services hitherto under the broad umbrella of the Department of Local Government and Public Health. In 1949, the first nursing advisor was appointed to the Department. The Health Acts of 1947 and 1953 provided a legislative basis for new developments. Some of them would have a marked impact on community nursing services. The new statutory provisions included the introduction of midwifery and infant welfare services up to the age of six weeks; and there was considerable emphasis on the preventive and treatment aspects of child health in general. During 1958 the Minister for Health introduced the title "public health nurse" in substitution for the title "district nurse" then used by health authorities. The activities of the voluntary nursing bodies, the Queen's Institute and the Lady Dudley Scheme, were phased out and gradually integrated with the services of the statutory authorities. The concept of the public health nurse became the subject of considerable discussion and her role more clearly formulated, culminating in a ministerial circular during 1966 which prescribed wide-ranging responsibilities including assisting at clinics and dispensaries, child welfare and school health examinations, domiciliary nursing and, where required, domiciliary midwifery. (In the meantime a full-time five month course of training in public health nursing had been initiated by An Bord Altranais during 1959/60. It became an annual event and was extended to six months and later to nine months. The numbers of participants in the courses varied annually but were as high as 116 in 1977).

Psychiatric Nursing

2.26   When the General Nursing Council of Ireland was established in 1919, among the classifications of nurses provided for on its register were those working in psychiatric nursing. Persons who already held the certificate of the Royal Medico-Psychological Association were granted automatic registration, but after 1935, admission to the register had to be through the Council's own examinations. Individual psychiatric hospitals had to be recognised as suitable training centres before candidates were accepted for examination: the trainees were recruited by each hospital. The change-over from hospitals staffed by untrained personnel to those having a full complement of professionally trained staff was a slow process and was completed only during the 1960's. However, progress had been accelerated as new treatments for mental illness were introduced in chemotherapy and psychotherapy requiring greater nursing skills. Along the way there were long-running negotiations between the unions concerned, the Department of Health and the health authorities leading to the establishment of parity of conditions between all the district mental hospitals and the improvement of pay and conditions generally. The psychiatric nurses became a strongly unionised profession, initially mainly under the aegis of the Irish Transport and General Worker's Union, joined subsequently by the Psychiatric Nurses Association. The issues of promotion on seniority and the integration of male and female nurses was the source of protracted difficulties between the Association and health service employers from the 1970's onwards.

2.27   In recent decades there has been a huge transformation in the pattern of services for persons with mental illness. At the end of December 1958 there were 21,046 patients residing in the district mental hospitals. By the end of 1995 the number had been reduced to 5,830 in all psychiatric hospitals and units. This radical change has come about as a result of various influences, but mainly due to the introduction of new treatments in chemotherapy and psychotherapy which reduced the need for residential care and enabled a great amount of mental illness to be dealt with outside the hospital setting. A notable change in the treatment of mental illness has been the increasing integration of services for the mentally and physically ill reflected by the inclusion of psychiatric units in the larger general hospitals.

Mental Handicap Nursing

2.28   Up to the 1950's there was relatively little provision for special services for persons with mental handicap. Stewarts Hospital was opened in 1869: the next special institution was not established until the Daughters of Charity inaugurated St. Vincent's Home, Cabra, in 1926. There was a long gap before further special accommodation was provided; many mentally handicapped persons were admitted to the district mental hospitals in the absence of any alternative provision for them. With the recognition by government policy of the shortcomings in existing services, there were considerable additions from the 1960's onwards by way of special residential and day centres for the handicapped. One of the first improvements made in the quality of the expanding services was the development of teachers trained in special education and it became increasingly obvious that the introduction of a body of nurses trained in mental handicap would enhance the services further. Hitherto, there were some staff members in the residential centres with a background in one of the other nursing disciplines but, as the numbers in residential care grew, there was increasing dependence on untrained assistants. Following an approach from the Department of Health, the Board accepted the need for a special training course and established a register for mental handicap nurses. The first training schools offering a three year course for nurses in mental handicap opened in 1959 at St. Joseph's (St. Louise's School), Clonsilla operated by the Daughters of Charity and at Drumcar, County Louth, under the aegis of the Brothers of St. John of God. A number of other schools followed. Subsequently, the school at Clonsilla became the national applications centre for all persons wishing to train in mental handicap nursing, but the selection process was carried out by the individual nursing schools. A revised syllabus was introduced in 1992.

Midwifery

2.29　　The practice of midwifery has changed radically since the mid-century, particularly since the years of the Second World War. As late as 1956, thirty-one percent of all births were home deliveries. But, influenced by the view of the health authorities and the medical profession that the safest place for a birth is in a maternity hospital or unit under obstetric management, domiciliary deliveries are now exceptional. During 1996, when there were 50,390 registered births in Ireland, only 206 of them were home births. In recent times a demand has been developing among some mothers and midwives for the greater recognition of home-based maternity services and of the role of the independent midwife.

The Second Phase of Regulation of the Profession

2.30　　With the development of the health services in the late 1940's, nursing expanded and became more specialised. New training needs emerged that were not being met. Nurses were also looking for more autonomy in decisions about their profession. The case was made for the integration of midwifery and nursing under the same regulatory body. The Government accepted the need to make changes to the arrangements for the regulation of the profession. The Nurses Act 1950, dissolved the General Nursing Council and the Central Midwives Board and replaced them by a single body, An Bord Altranais (The Nursing Board), established in June, 1951. For the first time nurses themselves were given a substantial voice in the regulation of their affairs. The new body consisted of a board of twenty three members, including twelve nurses elected by their own profession and six doctors drawn from designated specialities and general practice. Provision was made for a special midwives committee thus, for the first time, bringing into association the regulation of midwifery and other areas of nursing.

2.31　　During the 1950's the register consisted of nine divisions: - general, general (male), fever, sick children's, mental, sanatorium, tuberculosis (post-registration), orthopaedic (post-registration) and midwives. Between 1959 and 1974 a number of other divisions of the register were added: these were mental handicap, public health, advanced psychiatric, clinical teachers, nurse tutors and two divisions were closed: sanatorium and infectious diseases.

2.32　　In 1975, the Minister for Health established a Working Party on General Nursing to examine and report on the role of nurses in the health services, on the education, training and grading structures appropriate for that role in the future, and to make recommendations. The establishment of the Working Party was in response to discontent among nurses about the role of nurses in the health services and health service management and concern about the education and training of student nurses.

2.33　　The Working Party made wide ranging recommendations, including changes to the functions and operation of An Bord Altranais. In particular, it recommended the introduction of a live register of nurses with an annual retention fee, the appointment of a Fitness to Practise Committee and the notification of the Board by employers of serious misconduct by nurses. It also recommended a more consistent and policy oriented role for the Board in relation to schools of nursing. The Working Party reported in 1980.

2.34   The recommendations of the Working Party in relation to the role of the Board were included in the Nurses Act 1985. The Act has as its general concern the promotion of "high standards of professional education and training and professional conduct among nurses". Seventeen of the twenty nine members of the Board are elected by the profession, with the remainder appointed by the Minister for Health and Children.

2.35   Under the Act, a "nurse" is defined as a woman or a man whose name is entered in the register and includes a "midwife" and "nursing" includes "midwifery". A "midwife" is defined as a person whose name is entered in the midwives division of the register. Under rules made in accordance with that Act there are now seven divisions of the register, namely, general nursing, psychiatric nursing, mental handicap nursing, sick children's nursing, public health nursing, midwifery and registered nurse tutor.

2.36   *Changes in the Professional Role of Nurses in Ireland 1980 - 1997* (by Sarah Condell), is one of the literature reviews undertaken on behalf of the Commission. As mentioned in chapter one, this is published separately to the report and completes the history of the profession in Ireland to the present day.

The Future Direction of Nursing and Midwifery

Chapter 3

The Future Direction of Nursing and Midwifery

3.1   This chapter reflects on the high quality of Irish nursing which is illustrated by the level of public satisfaction with the service. The chapter outlines a future framework which will build on the existing status and reputation of Irish nursing and midwifery and provide a basis for the further development of the profession. A brief overview of nursing in Ireland is first presented followed by an overview of Patricia Benner's model of nursing skill acquisition, which reflects the richness and complexity of the practice of nursing. The Commission recognises that Benner's model represents just one view, of which there are many, on the practice of nursing.

A Brief Overview of Nursing in Ireland

3.2   By far the largest group of persons employed in the health services today are nurses. At the end of 1996, there was a total of 53,641 nurses recorded on the register (An Bord Altranais, 1996). Of these, 44,822 were on the active file and therefore were eligible to practise in this country. Of the total number registered at the end of 1996, ninety-three percent were female.

3.3   Qualifications registered on the active file in respect of each division of the register maintained by the Board at the end of 1996 were as follows:

Table 1	Number of qualifications registered on each division of the register (source An Bord Altranais Annual Report 1996)
Division	Number of Qualifications
General	36,243
Psychiatric	8,615
Sick Children's	2,821
Mental Handicap	2,865
Midwifery	12,136
Public Health	1,667
Tutor	331
Other	438
Total	**65,116**

3.4   The number of nurses employed by health boards and voluntary hospitals/agencies funded directly by the Department of Health at the end of December 1996 totalled 27,264. Of this number, sixty-five percent were at staff nurse grade. A further breakdown of these figures by employer shows:

Table 2 Number of nurses employed in the public health services in Ireland	
Total number of nurses employed by health boards	17,234
Total number of nurses employed by voluntary hospitals	7,886
Total number of nurses in voluntary mental handicap agencies	2,144
Total	**27,264***

This figure excludes nurses employed by voluntary health agencies funded by health boards.

3.5 Many nurses are employed in private hospitals, nursing homes and by nursing agencies. Others work as practice nurses with general practitioners. Some have chosen to work in the industrial/corporate sector while others have chosen to leave nursing altogether. Significant numbers of Irish nurses work overseas and have made a substantial contribution to the development of health services worldwide.

3.6 At the end of December 1996, the numbers in the main classifications of personnel in the public health services were:

Table 3 Number of nurses in context of all health care workers	
Management/Administration	8,151
Medical/Dental	4,684
Nursing	27,264
Paramedical	5,576
Support Service	18,461
Maintenance/Technical	1,618
Total	**65,755**

The above figures indicate the huge resource that nursing services are within the health service as a whole.

The Benner Model of Nursing Skill Acquisition

3.7 The practice of nursing requires a combination of technical and caring skills. It has often been suggested that it is sometimes difficult to characterise the qualities that underpin high quality nursing care. Ellen Savage, in the literature review entitled *An Examination of the Changes in the Professional Role of the Nurse Outside of Ireland*, examined international literature on the practice of nursing. The literature review considered international concepts of nursing practice and, in particular, considered the work of Patricia Benner which, as stated previously, captures the richness and complexity of nursing practice. The concepts developed by Patricia Benner in relation to nursing apply equally to midwifery. Nursing practice does not remain static following the registration of a nurse; rather through experience and further education, nurses develop their skills.

3.8 Benner (1984, 1996) through in-depth interviewing and observations, identified that nurses pass through five levels of skill performance in clinical practice. These are characterised as; novice practice, advanced beginner practice, competent practice, proficient practice and expert practice. Experience was seen as the critical element in the progression of a nurse through the levels of practice.

Novice Practice

A novice practitioner is characterised as being reliant on objective rules and facts and direct instruction to guide action. The practitioner is inexperienced and does not demonstrate the ability to prioritise work.

Advanced Beginner Practice

Practitioners at this level develop a greater self awareness as a nurse and become less reliant on rules, facts and direct instruction and are more context free in their practice. However, they are aware of the limitations of their practice and therefore seek advice and assistance from more experienced nurses who act as role models.

Competent Practice

A practitioner at this level of practice is characterised by a sense of role mastery and an ability to cope and manage many contingencies of clinical nursing. Practice at this level is planned and evolves on the basis of long-term goals and prioritisation.

Proficient Practice

Practice at this level is based on a holistic and deep understanding of situations. The hallmarks of proficient practice are increased perceptual acuity, responsiveness to particular situations and requires an experiential base with a particular client group. The clinical skills of a nurse at this level of practice depend on a perceptual grasp of qualitative distinctions, which can only be acquired by seeing and contrasting many similar and distinct clinical situations over time.

Expert Practice

The expert practitioner is characterised by an intuitive grasp of the most salient aspect of each situation with the minimum number of cues and such practice is based on a large reserve of experience. Unlike the proficient level, there is no detached decision making, deliberation or contemplation at this stage. Clinical grasp is inextricably linked with clinical response. Expert practice represents the essence of clinical judgement and is the pinnacle of clinical performance from the most knowledgeable members of the profession.

3.9 Benner's theory has been used to theoretically underpin clinical career pathways in some countries. However, the concept of skill progression applies equally to staff nurses, many of whom can be characterised as expert practitioners. It reflects the progression of nursing practice and recognises the concept, not unique to nursing, that there are different levels of practice-based on experience and education. The Commission outlines its proposals on a clinical career pathway in chapter six of this report. The theory reflects the complexity of nursing practice and is equally applicable to all disciplines. Nursing practice is constantly developing and represents a unique and crucial interaction with patients or clients. The type of interaction that takes place is often determined by the area of nursing activity and reflects the particular characteristics of each discipline.

3.10 The World Health Organisation (WHO) in 1996 stated that "the uniqueness of nursing lies in the ability of the nurse to combine all the activities of nursing practice in response to the needs of individuals, families and groups within differing situations and environments". While this statement encapsulates much of what nursing is, the Commission believes that the essence of Irish nursing extends beyond that and is inextricably linked with our Irish culture, embracing many of our values and norms.

3.11 In making recommendations for the future of nursing and midwifery in Ireland, the Commission is conscious that it is doing so in the context of world-wide change. Some of these changes are intrinsic to the profession, while others, although extrinsic, are equally influential. In acute general hospitals, trends such as shorter lengths of stay resulting in high patient turnover, have affected the acuity of patients being cared for. Subsequently, those being discharged to step-down facilities and into the community are increasingly more dependent, many requiring interventions that heretofore were only carried out in the domain of the acute hospital, for example, artificial feeding (via a percutaneous endoscopic gastrostomy tube). In the fields of psychiatry and mental handicap, the emphasis has shifted from institutionalisation to normalisation. In midwifery, the consumer movement has increasingly influenced the delivery of midwifery services. However, an unchanging feature of the profession is the focus on and concern in relation to the delivery of high quality care to patients and clients.

3.12 The Commission envisages that its recommendations will facilitate the development of the role of the nurse and the midwife and the sciences of nursing and midwifery in the rapidly changing health care environment mentioned above.

3.13 Throughout the consultative fora and in the written submissions, the Commission learned much about the profession's perception of itself and the issues involved in nursing and midwifery. As the Commission was established in response to recent industrial unrest, it is understandable that morale amongst nurses and midwives was at an all time low. However, with the establishment of the Commission, expectations rose, with the hope that many changes would ensue.

3.14 The Commission envisages that some of its recommendations will effect immediate change, while others will be implemented over a longer period.

3.15 The Commission wishes to stress from the outset that its recommendations will not be a panacea for all ills. Rather, structural changes will take place which will enable the profession to grow, while at the same time retain what is most cherished in Irish nurses and midwives, namely enthusiasm, energy, commitment, integrity, responsiveness to change, sense of humour, and above all, a deep sense of caring. Now is the time for nurses and midwives to gain independence through autonomy of practice and by shedding the facets of nursing and midwifery which have been perceived as restrictive and stunting the growth of the profession.

3.16 The Commission is of the opinion that the high esteem in which nurses and midwives are held in Ireland is something which needs to be emphasised and valued. In making any recommendations on the future of Irish nursing and midwifery, this ethos must be safeguarded.

3.17 As nursing and midwifery have long been regarded as an invisible art, the quality of nursing and midwifery services has been difficult to measure, compared with easily quantifiable issues such as costs. The Commission was anxious to measure the public's perception of nursing and midwifery and so decided to approach the Central Statistics Office (CSO) to seek their assistance.

3.18 The Commission is pleased to report that the first social topic to be included in the CSO, Quarterly National Household Survey was nursing care. The questions were designed to measure the public's level of contact with, and their assessment of, nursing services (see appendix four). A total of 33,500 households were included in the September to November 1997 quarterly survey and the results showed that forty-two percent of the population aged eighteen years or over had some contact with nursing services in the previous two years. Over ninety percent of respondents gave an overall rating of good or excellent to the nursing service they received (for detailed results see appendix five). These findings were similar to those of a survey undertaken by the Irish College of General Practitioners, when ninety-three percent of patients questioned held nurses in high regard (Irish Times, 06/05/98). The results of these two surveys are an affirmation of the high esteem in which Irish nurses are held.

3.19   As stated previously, Irish nurses enjoy a high standing and reputation not only in Ireland but internationally. The esteem in which nurses are held reflects the quality of their education and training. However, in a rapidly changing health service environment, the Commission considered the need to examine the preparation of students for entry to the profession. The Commission has sought to provide a framework which will prepare nurses to meet future health care needs into the next century. Changes in education will no doubt have an influence on shifting role boundaries.

3.20   The Commission acknowledges that for many years, nurses and midwives have been furthering their own education either through full-time study, distance learning courses or in-service training. This professional development has enabled nurses and midwives to cope more effectively with change. While some nurses and midwives have pursued their studies in a very structured way, with a clear vision of where they are going, others have undertaken further study without a sense of direction as to which pathway they wish to pursue. This may have been due to difficulty in accessing relevant courses or restrictive choices in courses available.

3.21   The Commission, in its recommendations, seeks to provide a framework which will give cohesion to further education for nurses and midwives by accrediting post-registration courses, taking account of standards of professional practice, geographical spread and access by nurses and midwives and in particular, service need.

3.22   The development of a clinical career pathway is seen as an important step for nurses wishing to remain in direct patient care, while at the same time advancing their own career. The Commission, in its recommendations, has sought to provide a framework for a clinical career pathway in nursing and midwifery which will have a beneficial impact on patient and client care whilst enhancing the role of the nurse or midwife. Nursing and midwifery in the future will be in partnership with patients, with a greater focus on health instead of on illness.

3.23   To date, the developments of diverse nursing and midwifery roles have been adhoc and reactive to change and have not occurred in a systematic way. This has led to shifting role boundaries and lack of a clear definition of the role of the nurse or midwife, resulting in overlap with other professions' roles which in turn can lead to conflict. On the other hand, rigid boundaries can be restrictive to practice and may in fact exacerbate conflict within the profession itself.

3.24   Nurses and midwives themselves acknowledge that there is a need to evaluate nursing critically as approaches to it change from the old mechanistic, but nevertheless effective way of task oriented nursing and midwifery, to a modern holistic and individualised style of patient care. Such critical analysis can only occur in the context of research and evidence-based practice. It is crucial to engender a culture of research and critical analysis to underpin practice which will improve patient care.

3.25   The scope of medical practice certainly impinges on the scope of nursing practice. The proposed changes by the Medical Council to the intern year and the deliberations of the recently established forum on medical manpower will have a bearing on the extended role of the nurse or midwife. It is against this background, where there is an examination of the future roles of other professionals in the health service, that nursing must examine its role. The Commission welcomes the recent initiative by An Bord Altranais to examine the parameters for the practice of nursing in its forthcoming review of the scope of practice.

3.26   Implementation of change will almost certainly be dependent on effective leaders and the Commission, in its recommendations on the role of the nurse and midwife in the management of services, acknowledges this.

3.27   In the context of the health service as a whole, the Commission envisages that nursing will be well represented at all levels of planning and decision making so that nurses will have a voice as health service policy develops.

3.28   The Commission is of the opinion that the nursing profession is able to assume greater responsibilities in self-regulation and develop further as an independent profession in the management of its own affairs. This will ensure that Irish nurses continue to be held in high regard and are recognised as a valuable resource to the health services.

Regulation of the
Nursing Profession

Chapter

4

Regulation of the Nursing Profession

4.1   Historically it appears that nursing has been regulated and supervised rather than self-regulating. While the Nurses Act 1985 provided for a greater degree of independence and self-regulation, the Commission considers that the process is not yet complete. The Commission considers that there is a need for the profession to assume greater responsibility for the development of the profession and to ensure professional leadership in nursing and midwifery.

4.2   ***The Commission recommends that the nursing profession take greater responsibility for the regulation and practice of the profession and for ensuring professional leadership in nursing and midwifery.*** The role of An Bord Altranais (the Board), as the profession's regulatory body, is critical to the achievement of greater responsibility and the promotion of professional leadership. For this reason, the Commission makes a number of important recommendations in relation to the Board.

4.3   This chapter outlines the current regulatory framework for the nursing profession in Ireland. The Commission was conscious of the need to examine the regulatory framework in light of the many educational and practice developments in nursing which have taken place in recent years. In addition, the Commission considered the regulatory framework in light of its recommendations on a revised future framework for pre-registration education, professional development and the management of nursing and midwifery.

The Nurses Act 1985

4.4   The legislation currently providing for the regulation of the nursing profession is the Nurses Act 1985 (the 1985 Act). As indicated in chapter two, the 1985 Act provided for the establishment of a new Board to provide for the regulation, control and education of nurses and other matters related to the practice of nursing. The main functions of the Board under the 1985 Act relate to:

- the maintenance of a register of nurses;

- the control of education and training of student nurses and the post-registration training of nurses;

- the operation of the fitness to practise procedures; and

- the ensuring of compliance with European Union directives on nursing and midwifery.

The Board has as its general concern under the 1985 Act, the promotion of "high standards of professional education and training and professional conduct among nurses". As part of its function the Board published a code of professional conduct for each nurse and midwife in 1988. The code was intended to provide a framework to assist nurses and midwives in making professional decisions, to carry out her or his responsibilities, and to promote high standards of professional conduct. The present board of An Bord Altranais consists of twenty-nine members, seventeen of whom are nurses elected by the nursing profession and the remainder are appointed by the Minister for Health and Children (the Minister) and are drawn from the medical profession, the management of the health services, education interests and the general public.

Fitness to Practise

4.5   The Board is required under the 1985 Act to establish a Fitness to Practise Committee, all of whom must be members of the Board, a majority must be elected members and one third must be non-elected members. The 1985 Act confers on the Board power to inquire into complaints against members of the nursing profession regarding their fitness to practise either for professional misconduct or because of physical or mental disability. The Board has power to remove or suspend the name of a nurse for a period or attach conditions to the retention of the name of a nurse on the register. There must then be an application to the High Court which may confirm, cancel or vary the decision of the Board. In addition, the Board may advise, admonish or censure persons in relation to professional conduct.

Other Legislation Relevant to the Practice of Nursing

4.6   The nursing profession also operates within the parameters of legislation other than the 1985 Act. In the area of professional practice these include the Misuse of Drugs Acts 1977 and 1984, the Health (Nursing Homes) Act 1990, the Child Care Act 1991, the Data Protection Act 1988 and the Freedom of Information Act 1997. In addition, nurses need to be conscious of developments in the law in the area of negligence.

4.7   The Misuse of Drugs Acts set out detailed provisions on the storage, dispensing and administration of controlled drugs. Controlled drugs comprise scheduled and dangerous drugs. It is a criminal offence to be in breach of the Misuse of Drugs Acts. The Board also issued a document - *Guidance to Nurses and Midwives on the Administration of Medical Preparations* - to assist nurses in relation to the administration of medical preparations, the fourth edition of which was published in 1997.

4.8   The Health (Nursing Homes) Act 1990 updated the law on nursing homes with the aim of ensuring high standards of care. Under this Act a new framework was put in place for the exercise of responsibilities by nurses working in nursing homes. The Child Care Act 1991 updated the law on the protection of children and places certain statutory obligations on those health care workers working or in contact with children. This Act has particular importance for public health nurses working with families in the community. Nurses need to be cognisant of the Data Protection Act 1988 when dealing with issues on the confidentiality of computerised patient records and of the implications of the Freedom of Information Act 1997 when also dealing with patient records.

Issues Arising from the Consultative Process

4.9   As indicated above, nursing and midwifery practice is regulated by a combination of a statutory professional regulatory body and legislation. The general framework is similar to that for the medical profession which has a statutory professional body and is also governed by other relevant legislation. A range of concerns in relation to the current regulatory framework was identified during the consultative process undertaken by the Commission. These concerns related primarily to the perceived lack of professional guidance and leadership from the regulatory body, together with a perceived lack of independence and what was viewed as a very punitive and cumbersome fitness to practise procedure.

4.10   There was a view expressed by nurses and midwives, in submissions and at the workshops and seminars organised by the Commission, that the Board was not being sufficiently pro-active in leading the development of nursing and midwifery practice. It was also suggested that the Board appeared to constrain practice in some areas and offered little guidance in other areas. Nurses and midwives were concerned about extending the parameters of professional practice in the absence of clear guidance from their regulatory body. There were concerns that if professional issues were unclear now or in the future, nurses and midwives seeking to extend their practice could face investigation before the Fitness to Practise Committee. It was suggested during the consultative process that the Board should empower nurses and midwives to a much greater extent to make professional decisions, rather than have narrowly focused prescriptive guidelines in certain areas. There was a view that in recent years the Board has constrained the development of nursing and midwifery practice, rather than assist nurses and midwives to develop safely the parameters of their practice. In their submission to the Commission, the Board recognised the wish of nurses and midwives to extend the parameters of their professional practice and their wish for a distinct role with greater autonomy, responsibility and accountability.

4.11   Concerns were also raised about what was seen as the lack of independence of the Board. The view was put forward during the consultative process that the Board was not sufficiently independent of the Department of Health and Children and nursing trade unions. There were some complaints in relation to the presence of representatives of the Department of Health and Children, health service management and medical practitioners on the professional regulatory body for nurses and midwives. It was noted that there were no similar representatives on the professional regulatory body for medical practitioners. The lack of perceived independence appeared to create an impression that the "real" decisions on issues before the Board were taken elsewhere.

A Future Framework for the Regulation of the Nursing Profession

4.12   The Commission, in considering the views expressed during the consultative process, examined the regulatory framework for other professional bodies in Ireland. There is a need to give the Board a more clearly defined professional focus and distinct identity. There is also the need to give nurses and midwives a greater sense of ownership and inclusion in its decision making process and activities. The Board has already begun to address some of the concerns expressed during the consultative process and the first public meeting of the Board took place on 11 June, 1998. However, there is a need to amend the legislative framework (the 1985 Act) underpinning the Board, in order to allow for certain structural reforms. In view of the necessity to introduce reforms as quickly as possible, the Commission does not recommend a new consolidation Act, but rather an amendment of the 1985 Act. *The Commission recommends that the profession take greater control over its own destiny through ownership of the Board.*

The General Concern of An Bord Altranais

4.13   In addressing the need to provide a clearer professional regulatory focus to the activities of the Board, the Commission considers that the protection of the public should be made explicit as a general concern. The making explicit of the protection of the public was requested by the Board in its submission to the Commission and is in keeping with national and international developments in relation to professional regulatory bodies. Irish nurses and midwives have an international reputation for their high standards of education, training, practice and professional conduct. The maintenance and development of these standards through the activities of the Board will ensure that the Irish public will continue to enjoy the highest standard of nursing and midwifery care. *The Commission therefore recommends that section 6(1) of the 1985 Act be amended to provide that the general concern of the Board shall be the protection of the public through the promotion of high standards of professional education, training and practice and professional conduct among nurses and midwives.*

The Scope of Professional Practice

4.14   As indicated earlier, a major concern voiced by nurses during the consultative process was the perception that the Board was not sufficiently proactive in providing professional support and guidance. This concern related in particular to the view that the Board was constraining practice, rather than allowing nurses and midwives the flexibility to develop their practice safely, in the rapidly developing health service environment. The absence of a document for Irish nurses similar to *The Scope of Professional Practice* (1992) in the United Kingdom was identified in the Interim Report of the Commission. It is acknowledged that the Board intends to undertake a project to examine the scope of practice in Irish nursing and midwifery. However, the Commission considers that there is a need for the Board to provide greater professional leadership for the nursing profession and create a framework which would enable nurses and midwives to develop their practice within safe parameters. It is necessary that the legislation providing for the role of the Board reflects the focus on professional leadership. ***Therefore, the Commission recommends that section 51(2) of the 1985 Act be amended to provide that it shall be a function of the Board to give professional guidance and support on matters relating to clinical practice as well as giving guidance on all matters relating to ethical conduct and behaviour.***

Limited Prescribing

4.15   Many midwives during the consultative process recounted situations in which nurses or midwives might need to administer non-prescribed drugs or medicated dressings in the interests of the patient, in the absence of medical support. The Commission considers that there is a need to allow greater flexibility to nurses and midwives in the administration of non-prescribed drugs according to agreed protocols with medical practitioners. ***Therefore, the Commission recommends that the Board as a matter of urgency, review the guidelines in relation to the administration or application of non-prescribed drugs by nurses and midwives***.

4.16   The Commission received a number of submissions from pharmacists in relation to the Medical Products (Prescription and Control of Supply) Regulations 1996. It was stated that these regulations provide, for the first time in law, a specific entitlement for nurses to supply medicinal products in the course of a service provided by a hospital or supply medicinal products in a quantity sufficient for a period of treatment not exceeding three days, in the course of a service provided by a hospital delivering community mental health services to patients. It was suggested in submissions from pharmacists that nurses were not sufficiently competent to carry out the functions allowed to them under the regulations. The Commission was of the view that the criticism by pharmacists of statutory provisions governing the administration of drugs was not a matter for its consideration.

Membership of An Bord Altranais

4.17   Section 9 of the 1985 Act provides for the membership on the Board. The section provides for a membership of seventeen nurses elected by the nursing profession and twelve persons appointed by the Minister. The elected membership consists of five nurses engaged in training nurses (representing general nursing, sick children's nursing, psychiatric nursing, mental handicap nursing and midwifery), five nurses engaged in nursing administration (representing general nursing, sick children's nursing, psychiatric nursing, mental handicap nursing and midwifery) and seven nurses engaged in clinical nursing practice (two of whom represent general nursing, two of whom represent psychiatric nursing and one representative each from public health nursing, mental handicap nursing and midwifery). The Minister appoints twelve members to the Board, three of whom are registered medical practitioners, two representatives of health service management, two representatives of the Department of Health, one representative of third-level education establishments, one person experienced in the field of education, one nurse and two persons to represent the interest of the general public. The board holds office for a period of five years.

4.18   The Commission considers that there is a need to provide for a more distinct identity to the professional regulatory authority for the nursing profession. The consultative process clearly identified that nurses and midwives did not have a sense of ownership of the Board. A need was identified for greater transparency and accountability in its operation. The lack of a sense of ownership amongst nurses and midwives and concerns in relation to the perceived secrecy of the operation of the Board must be of major concern to a professional regulatory body which is charged with the protection of the public through the promotion of high standards in nursing and midwifery. If nurses and midwives perceive the Board as not being adequately representative of the profession and as merely an organisation to take punitive action against nurses and midwives, then it will not have sufficient standing in the profession to perform its important functions.

4.19   In order to define more clearly the role of the Board and to provide nurses and midwives with a greater sense of identity with it, the Commission considers that in future, the membership of the Board should consist only of elected members of the profession together with representatives of the public interest appointed by the Minister and certain other categories of person co-opted by the Board. There is also a need to raise the profile of sick children's nursing and the Commission therefore considers that there is a need to increase the representation from that discipline on the Board. Similarly in the interests of equity, the Commission considers that the representation of public health nursing on the Board should also be increased. Nursing in care of the elderly is an increasingly important area of nursing activity. The ageing profile of the Irish population presents many challenges to the health services and nursing in particular. Nursing in care of the elderly settings is considered in greater detail in chapter nine of the report. However, the Commission considers that one of the representatives of clinical practice in general nursing should be specified as representing general nurses in clinical practice in care of the elderly. The representation of the public interest should be increased to three members who will have a very important function in representing the interests of patients and clients of the health service. In the past, some representatives of the public interest have also been former nurses. Given their role on the Board, the Commission considers the appointment of nurses or former nurses to represent the public interest as inappropriate.

4.20   Future Boards may decide, that in addition to the elected membership and representation of the public interest, there may be a need for expertise or a perspective not represented on the Board to be available to it. The Commission therefore considers that future Boards should be enabled to co-opt additional members to the Board. It is important that this power to co-opt is not used as a mechanism to bring candidates who were unsuccessful in elections onto the Board. Its focus should be entirely on bringing additional expertise or alternative perspectives to the membership of the Board. The Commission considers that the category of person who may be co-opted to the board be confined in amending legislation to the following categories; representatives of any areas of the health services, or of nursing education, or of a category of nursing not elected to the board. Not more than four persons should be co-opted to the Board.

4.21   **The Commission recommends that the 1985 Act be amended to provide that the Board shall consist of a maximum of twenty-eight members appointed in the following way:**

        (a) eight nurses resident in the State, three of whom are representative of nurses engaged in clinical practice in general nursing (one of whom shall be working in care of the elderly), two of whom are representative of nurses engaged in clinical practice in psychiatric nursing and three of whom are nurses engaged in clinical practice in each of the following disciplines, sick children's, mental handicap and public health nursing, respectively, elected by nurses;

(b) *five nurses resident in the State who are engaged in nursing education in each of the following disciplines, general, sick children's, psychiatric, mental handicap and public health, respectively, elected by nurses;*

(c) *five nurses resident in the State who are engaged in nursing management in each of the following disciplines, general, sick children's, psychiatric, mental handicap and public health, respectively, elected by nurses;*

(d) *three midwives resident in the State, one of whom is engaged in midwifery education, one of whom is engaged in midwifery management and one of whom is engaged in clinical practice, elected by midwives;*

(e) *three persons appointed by the Minister, representative of the interests of the general public, who are not nurses or former nurses; and*

(f) *not more than four persons (other than candidates unsuccessful in elections to the Board) nominated by the Board at its discretion and appointed by the Minister, representative of any areas of the health services or of nursing education or of a category of nursing not elected to the Board.*

4.22   The Commission considers that given the central role of the Board to the development of nursing and midwifery there should be a continuity of membership between the terms of office of boards. ***Therefore the Commission recommends that the 1985 Act be amended to provide that the term of office for members of the Board be of six years duration with half the number going out of office every three years.*** This would mean having elections more often but would ensure that some continuity was maintained in the Board. The co-opted members would go out of office at the same time as elected and appointed members of the Board. The initial co-option of additional members should take cognisance of half the Board going out of office after three years. The Commission considers that the provisions in the Second Schedule of the 1985 Act, limiting membership of the Board to two consecutive terms and for filling casual vacancies, either by co-option by the Board in the case of elected or co-opted members, or by the Minister in the case of appointed members, should continue to apply. The rule of tenure limiting membership of the Board to two consecutive terms should not apply to the Chief Nursing Officer of the Department of Health and Children, if co-opted to the Board.

4.23   Those members who go out of office at the first election at the end of three years could be determined in the following way:

(i)   of the members concerned with nurse training, the representatives of sick children's, psychiatric and public health nursing go out of office;

(ii)   of the members concerned with nursing and midwifery management, the representatives of mental handicap and general nursing and midwifery go out of office;

(iii) of the members concerned with clinical nursing, the representatives of mental handicap and public health nursing, one of the two psychiatric nurses, and one of the three general nurses go out of office;

(iv)   of the three persons appointed by the Minister, two (chosen by lot) go out of office at the end of three years; and

(v)   of the persons co-opted by the Board, one half (as decided by the Board) shall go out of office at the end of three years.

The remaining elected, appointed or co-opted members go out of office at the end of six years.

The Commission also recommends that section 10 of the 1985 Act be amended to provide a new sub-section providing that the appointment of members to the Board by the Minister shall be made within eight weeks of notice to him of the necessity to make such appointments.

4.24 The Commission is of the view that the Board has a different remit to the nursing trade unions whose focus is different. It is essential that the Board is seen as independent of both the Department of Health and Children and the nursing trade unions. Industrial relations are not the concern of a professional regulatory body and it is important that the Board maintains a distinct professional focus. Members of the Board should bring an independent professional perspective and the status of the Board will be undermined if members are generally viewed as delegates of other organisations.

4.25 The low turnout amongst nurses and midwives in elections to the Board in recent years was identified as a source of concern within the profession. In the elections to the Board in 1997 the number of nurses and midwives eligible to vote was 40,466 of whom 9,417 (twenty-three percent) returned ballot papers. The problem of getting voting response at election time was considered by the Commission. It would be important to get a good voter turn-out for elections so that the Board would "belong" to the electorate. Methods of improving the turnout amongst nurses and midwives were considered and *the Commission recommends that the Board*:

- *profile all candidates in the Board newsletter with a view to affording each candidate an equal opportunity;*

- *provide a free copy of the register for all candidates;*

- *investigate how to encourage nurses and midwives to run as candidates;*

- *continue to allow nurses and midwives attend meetings of the board, so that they will become familiar with the work of the Board; and*

- *simplify the voting system (this might include "Freepost" return of ballot paper and the provision of swipe cards (complete with PIN number) to facilitate completion of the ballot paper).*

Committees Other Than Fitness to Practise

4.26 The Board has power under Section 13 of the 1985 Act to establish committees to perform functions which may better or more conveniently be performed by committees with non board members on them, though the Chair must be a Board member. Each committee may establish its own procedures subject to direction from the Board. *The Commission recommends that the Board consider the more active use of section 13 of the 1985 Act to broaden even further the range of expertise available to it in considering issues of concern to the profession.*

Fitness to Practise

4.27 The number of members on the Fitness to Practise Committee is not laid down by the 1985 Act. However, the Commission understands that the number of members on the current Fitness to Practise Committee is fourteen. The 1985 Act specifies that:

(i) members must all be members of the board;

(ii)   the Chair must not be the President or the Vice-President; and

(iii)   the majority must be elected members and at least one third must be non elected.

The committee enquires into:

(a)   alleged professional misconduct; or

(b)   alleged unfitness to engage in practice by reason of physical or mental disability.

The committee can inform the Board if in its opinion there is not sufficient cause and the Board then decides whether or not to go ahead with an inquiry.

Current Fitness to Practise Procedures

4.28   If the Fitness to Practise Committee considers there is sufficient cause or is so directed by the Board, it holds an enquiry. The subject of the enquiry is given notice of evidence and the opportunity to be present with representatives. The Chief Executive Officer (or another) presents the evidence. On completion, the committee presents a report of the findings to the Board, specifying the nature of the allegations, the evidence and other relevant matters and its opinion on the allegations on the health issue or misconduct. Subject to the regulations of the Board and the 1985 Act, the committee may regulate its own procedure. The Board makes a decision on the report of the committee.

4.29   While all members of the Fitness to Practise Committee are entitled to participate in an enquiry, according to the rules of the committee (signed on 25th September, 1997) the quorum is five, including the Chair. A two-thirds majority of those attending and entitled to vote is necessary for an adverse finding. At least one member of the committee shall be from the specialist field in which the nurse is practising. The enquiry cannot continue in the absence of such a member without the consent of the nurse.

4.30   Under the present arrangements where a person has been found guilty by the Fitness to Practise Committee of professional misconduct or unfit to practise because of physical or mental disability, the full Board may decide that the name of the person should be erased or suspended from the register or retained subject to conditions. Notice of this decision must be sent forthwith to the person affected. She or he has twenty-one days beginning on the date of the decision to apply to the High Court for cancellation of such a decision.

4.31   If the person applies, the High Court may cancel the decision or declare it was proper for the Board to make such a decision and direct the erasure or suspension from the register for a specified period or give such other directions as the court thinks fit. Where a person applies and the Board satisfies the court that the person has delayed unduly in proceeding with the application, the court may, unless it sees good reason to the contrary, make similar decisions {Section 39(1), (2) and (3) of the 1985 Act}. If the person affected fails to apply to the High Court within twenty-one days, the Board may apply to the High Court for confirmation of a decision to erase or suspend a person from the register. The Court may confirm the decision unless it sees good reason to the contrary {Section 39(4) of the 1985 Act}.

A Revised Framework for Fitness to Practise

4.32   The Commission considered that a revised fitness to practise procedure was required, in particular to provide a more expeditious mechanism enabling preliminary enquiries into complaints and to distinguish between cases of professional misconduct and those where professional conduct may have been impaired by reason of ill-health. The Commission examined the United Kingdom Central

Council for Nursing, Midwifery and Health Visiting (UKCC) method of enquiries. The enquiry system there depends on whether it is a health issue or a misconduct issue. *The Commission recommends adopting a simplified version and that the 1985 Act be amended to provide for the following revised fitness to practise procedures. The revised framework provides for the setting up of three adhoc sub-committees drawn from the membership of the Fitness to Practise Committee. A person should not be a member of more than one sub-committee dealing with the same complaint(s) under the revised fitness to practise procedures.*

Preliminary Screening Sub-Committee

4.33   *The Commission recommends that there should be an ad hoc preliminary screening sub-committee, composed of three members of the Fitness to Practise Committee.* There should be no delay in bringing a complaint to the attention of the preliminary screening sub-committee, which would be expected to commence dealing with it within fourteen days of receipt of a complaint. If in the opinion of the preliminary screening sub-committee there is no prima facie case, the sub-committee reports to the Board, who can direct a hearing before either the health or professional conduct sub-committees or accept that there is no case to answer, in which case the complainant and the nurse are both informed and given the reasons. Those three members do not take part in any further steps in the case at Fitness to Practise Committee level. If there is a prima facie case, the matter is sent either to a health sub-committee if it is a health issue or to a professional conduct sub-committee if it is alleged misconduct.

Health Sub-Committee

4.34   *If a complaint relates to a health issue, the Commission recommends that there should be an ad hoc health sub-committee, composed of five members of the Fitness to Practise Committee (one of whom must be a representative of the public interest) to investigate the issue.* The nurse or midwife should be invited to be examined by two medical practitioners (paid for by the Board) from a panel set up by the Fitness to Practise Committee. These report to the health sub-committee. The nurse or midwife should also have the option of being examined by her or his own medical practitioner who may submit a report. The health sub-committee will consider if the issue of ill-health is proven or not and report to the board with recommendations. The aim of the health sub-committee should be to establish if the fitness to practise of the nurse or midwife is so impaired that the nurse or midwife is likely to be a danger to the public. The quorum for the sub-committee should be three. If ill-health is not proven and the Board considers there is an outstanding issue of misconduct, it is referred to the professional conduct sub-committee.

Professional Conduct Sub-Committee

4.35   *If a complaint relates to a misconduct issue, the Commission recommends that there should be an ad hoc professional conduct sub-committee, composed of five members of the Fitness to Practise Committee (one of whom must be a representative of the public interest and one of whom must be of the same discipline as the nurse) to investigate the issue.* The five members of the professional conduct sub-committee should differ from those appointed to the health sub-committee, if such a sub-committee examined the case previously. The professional conduct sub-committee considers if the complaint is proven and reports to the Board with recommendations. If a case which is prima facie dealing with misconduct, turns out to be a health issue, the Board may refer the matter to the health sub-committee to decide this issue (again the members of the health sub-committee should not have been members of the professional conduct sub-committee which previously examined the case). The quorum for the professional conduct sub-committee should be three.

4.36 The number of cases per annum is not large, so a preliminary screening sub-committee, health sub-committee or professional conduct sub-committee drawn from the Fitness to Practise Committee can be set up ad hoc by the Chair of the Committee depending on the availability of members for attendance at an enquiry. The aim should be to have a quick and fair resolution to allegations of unfitness to practise. The matter should not be delayed if a member has to drop out of an enquiry but it can continue provided there is a quorum. There would be an exception in the case where there is no member of the same discipline in a misconduct case unless with the consent of the nurse.

4.37 The suggested changes would require amendment of the 1985 Act by deleting the requirement that one third of the Fitness to Practise Committee should be appointed members and by making consequential changes to allow for the setting up of preliminary screening sub-committees, health sub-committees and professional conduct sub-committees instead of the full Fitness to Practise Committee. All the sub-committees would be constituted on an ad hoc basis from the membership of the Fitness to Practise Committee by the Chair of that committee, as required. The Commission makes a separate recommendation at paragraph 4.45 of this chapter in relation to allegations of misconduct against midwives.

Other Matters Relating to Fitness to Practise

4.38 If a nurse or midwife is convicted of an indictable offence (i.e. an offence warranting trial by jury in the Circuit or Central Criminal Court) within the State or the equivalent outside the State, his or her name may be erased from the register by the Board. The Commission considers this provision to be somewhat inflexible. Depending on the circumstances of each individual case, some lesser sanction may be more appropriate. ***The Commission recommends that section 42(1) of the 1985 Act be amended to extend the full range of sanctions to cases of conviction for an indictable offence.*** There should also be clarification of the procedure under this section so that the conviction can be proven by a certificate of conviction from the appropriate court and providing for the opportunity for the nurse or midwife to be heard in mitigation.

4.39 ***The Commission recommends that the 1985 Act be amended to allow for a sanction to be imposed by agreement between the nurse or midwife and the Board.*** Such a provision would allow for a compromise solution without the necessity of having or completing a full enquiry. However, the complainant should first be informed and given an opportunity to be heard in the interests of transparency.

4.40 The Board, in a submission to the Commission, sought a contribution by the State for the expenses of the Fitness to Practise hearings, on the basis that they concerned the protection of the public and also full reimbursement, if an application is made under Section 44 of the 1985 Act for an Interim Order for the protection of the public. The Commission does not support this view. An independent profession should bear the expenses of "policing" its own members and ensuring high standards of practice. However, if the Board is named as a defendant in a test case relating to the constitutionality of the 1985 Act (as amended) the Commission recommends that the State makes a contribution or pays the legal expenses of the Board involved in such a case.

4.41 At present the period within which a nurse or midwife may apply to the High Court for cancellation of a decision of the Board is twenty-one days from the date of the decision. ***The Commission recommends that section 39 of the 1985 Act be amended to allow a nurse*** *or midwife twenty-one days from the date of service of notification of a decision to apply to the High Court for cancellation of such a decision. The revised time period should also apply in relation to an application to the High Court by the Board for confirmation of a sanction.* The Commission does not recommend any other change in the fitness to practise procedure once the Board has made a decision to impose a sanction on a nurse or midwife and where there is no agreement between the parties on the sanction to be applied. The current requirement for application to the High Court to confirm its decision would remain, so that the Order which is final and binding is made by the court in the administration of justice and in accordance with the Constitution.

4.42   However, in the case where agreement is reached between the Board and the nurse or midwife, as to the sanction to be imposed, the Commission considers that an application to the High Court should not be necessary. *The Commission recommends that the 1985 Act be amended to remove the requirement of application to the High Court where the Board and nurse or midwife have reached agreement on the sanction to be imposed.*

4.43   *The Commission recommends that any sanction, other than a sanction pursuant to section 41 of the 1985 Act imposed against a person under the fitness to practise procedures, should be entered forthwith on the register against the name of the person for the duration of the sanction. The register should be open to inspection by members of the public.* A sanction imposed pursuant to section 41 of the 1985 Act, which allows the Board to advise, admonish or censure a nurse, should not be entered against the name of a person on the register.

Regulation of Midwifery

4.44   The Commission received numerous submissions from midwives that their distinct identity required explicit acknowledgement in any amending legislation. *The Commission acknowledges the request from midwives for recognition of their distinct identity and recommends that the title of the amending legislation should be the Nurses and Midwives Act.* The midwives complain with some justification that they have been written out and become invisible because of the provision in the interpretation section that "nurse" includes a "midwife". This provision is understandable from a drafting point of view as otherwise every time the word "nurse" is used, the word "midwife" would also have to be added. In the United Kingdom legislation they mention both nurses and midwives throughout the relevant Act. If it is feasible, the 1985 Act should be amended so that the definition is amended throughout the Act. If this is not possible, then in any future new consolidating Act, consideration should be given either to mentioning both nurses and midwives throughout the text or else separating the definitions of nurses and midwives so that there is no provision that the word "nurse" includes "midwife". It is a small point but it is one which causes a lot of resentment.

4.45   Midwives, in submissions to the Commission, requested the establishment of a statutory midwives committee. Such a committee existed prior to the 1985 Act and was requested as necessary to give practical expression to the distinct concerns and requirements of midwives. It was suggested that midwives, in caring for the needs of women during the course of pregnancy and following birth, had different concerns and needs to nurses. *The Commission* accepts these views and *recommends the 1985 Act be amended to provide for the restoration of a separate statutory midwives committee consisting of eight members. It is recommended that such a committee consist of the three elected midwife members of the Board and five registered midwives appointed by the Board. In light of the increasing demand for domiciliary midwifery services, it is recommended that one of the five registered midwives appointed by the Board should be a midwife currently engaged in providing domiciliary midwifery services. This committee should have power to draft the scope of practice for midwives subject to approval of the Board. In the case of an allegation of professional misconduct against a midwife, four of the midwives committee plus one member of the Fitness to Practise Committee, representative of the interests of the general public, should be constituted by the Chair of the Fitness to Practise Committee as a professional conduct sub-committee reporting back to the Board with recommendations. At least one of the midwives on the professional conduct sub-committee should be an elected member of the Board. Health cases can be heard by a health sub-committee appointed in the normal way by the Chair of the Fitness to Practise Committee.* Subject to the midwives professional conduct sub-committee, all other fitness to practise procedures would apply.

Registration

4.46 The Board in a submission to the Commission requested a new provision to enable a nurse or midwife to apply to delete her or his name (as in Medical Practitioners Act 1978). **The Commission** accepts this suggestion and **recommends that the 1985 Act be amended to provide that a nurse or midwife may apply to have her or his name removed from the register as is provided in section 33 of the Medical Practitioners Act 1978.**

4.47 It was suggested during the consultative process that the 1985 Act be amended to change from registration and retention of name on payment of an annual fee to a system of licensing on payment of a fee subject to satisfying the Board that a nurse/midwife continues to up-grade knowledge and skills through on-going education and training.

4.48 In the view of the Commission there is a difference in form but not in substance between a system of registration as opposed to a system of licensing. There is no basic difference between being entitled to practise because one's name is on a register and being entitled to practise because one has a licence. Also the issuing of licences would add another layer of work on top of actual registration which would have to be maintained.

4.49 The Board, in discussions with the Commission, expressed concerns in relation to the non-payment and late payment of retention fees by some nurses and midwives. The Commission accepts that it is not in the interests of the profession that some nurses and midwives do not contribute to maintaining the independent professional regulatory body. Under the 1985 Act, the procedure necessary for deleting a name from the register for non-payment of the retention fee is the same as for professional misconduct or unfitness to practise because of physical or mental disability. This entails an application to the High Court as outlined in paragraphs 4.30 and 4.31. The Commission considers that this procedure is unnecessarily cumbersome and should be changed. A system similar to that operated by veterinary surgeons should be adopted. **The Commission, therefore recommends that sub-paragraph (b) of section 39(1) of the 1985 Act be deleted (thus removing non-payment of the retention fee from the fitness to practise procedure) and that part III of the 1985 Act (dealing with registration) be amended to provide that after notice is given to the address on the register, the names of nurses or midwives who fail to pay the annual retention fee within the time provided by the rules, may be deleted from the register at any meeting of the Board after such time has expired. Notice of such a deletion is sent to the nurse or midwife involved, and the name can be restored to the register on application, on payment of a penalty fee. The rules should provide that the period within which the retention fee must be paid is from 1st January to 30th April in each year.** Nurses and midwives should be aware that if they fail

4

to pay the retention fee and consequently have their names deleted from the register, they will be liable under section 49(1)(a) of the 1985 Act which prohibits the use of the title of nurse or midwife by a person not on the register. If they use the name or title of nurse or midwife and are not on the register, they will be guilty of an offence.

4.50 The Commission supports the need of ensuring safe practice by all nurses and midwives. At present there is no general requirement by the Board for nurses or midwives who have not being practising for a considerable period of time to undergo a back to nursing or midwifery course. However, there is a requirement by the Board for nurses and midwives who have trained and worked abroad, but have not practised for three out of the preceding five years and wish to register here, to provide evidence of having satisfactorily completed such a course. This is to fulfil EU Directives 77/452 and 77/453 which deal with education requirements and freedom of movement respectively.

4.51 *The Commission recommends that the 1985 Act be amended to entitle the Board to require any nurse or midwife to satisfy it as to her or his relevant competencies, failing which the Board could require an up-date on skills and knowledge, as a condition of retention of name on the register, provided the purpose would be for the protection of the public even in the absence of any complaint.* This should get over any conflict between constitutional rights, as the right of the public to expect and get safe practice would probably be considered superior to the right of a nurse or midwife to work once registered. This would, however, be subject to confirmation by the Attorney General. Concern was expressed that this power could be abused and used as a threat for an ulterior motive against nurses. Therefore, it is important to ensure that this would not happen. *Rules for the exercise of this power, which are fair and equitable, would have to be drawn up by the Board and monitored to ensure that the concerns expressed about its exercise would not be realised.* (Des Kavanagh did not support this recommendation).

4.52 In submissions to the Commission, a number of nurses and midwives requested that additional qualifications and information be recorded on the register maintained by the Board. It was further suggested that the lack of information currently recorded on the register meant it was not a useful aid in workforce planning. The Commission is aware that the Board approved a proposal in September 1997 to have approved post-registration qualifications and relevant academic awards recorded with registration details. In order to be recorded on the register, a course must satisfy certain criteria specified by the Board. The Commission makes further recommendations in relation to the approval of post-registration courses to be recorded on the register maintained by the Board in chapter six of this report. In the light of those, *the Commission recommends the Board keep the criteria for recording of post-registration qualifications under constant review.*

4.53 When paying the annual fee, each nurse and midwife should be obliged to give particulars of the name of the employer and position held as of the 1st January each year. At present, the name of the employer is given but there is no obligation on the nurse or midwife to keep the information up-to-date. *The Commission recommends that the rules of the Board should be amended to provide that on payment of the retention fee each year, every nurse and midwife should be obliged to give particulars of the name of the employer and the position held as of 1st January in each year, such information to appear on the register.*

Care Assistants and Other Non-Nursing Personnel

4.54 The issue of the regulation of care assistants and other non-nursing personnel was raised in submissions and in workshops during the consultative process undertaken by the Commission. The increasing need for personnel to perform non-nursing tasks which had previously been carried out by nurses has resulted in an increasing number of care assistants and other non-nursing personnel in recent years. Concerns have been raised about the lack of standard qualifications and training for such personnel which raises issues in relation to the protection of the public and quality of care. In a submission to the Commission, the Board sought the deletion of section 30 of the 1985 Act which provides for registration by the Board of persons engaged in a profession or calling ancillary to nursing, because this is not part of the registration of nurses. It is considered that this section is intended to apply to care assistants.

4.55   The Commission agrees that the Board should not be involved in the registration of care assistants and other non-nursing personnel. The question immediately arises whether such personnel could be removed from a register and on what grounds. A register would give the impression of a two tier nursing system and result in public confusion in relation to the parameters of activity of nurses and care assistants. The Commission considers the control of non-nursing personnel as being an employers or employment issue. The Commission agrees that there needs to be a basic training curriculum with a range of courses. It is essential that nurses should be involved in this training so that appropriate standards are achieved. At present such training varies from place to place. The assistants will be working with and under the supervision of nurse. While section 30 of the 1985 Act is dormant and is unlikely to be activated, a call to repeal it would emphasise the necessity for providing adequate training. ***The Commission recommends that section 30 of the 1985 Act be deleted. The Commission also recommends that the Minister establish a working party comprised of representatives of the Department of Health and Children, the Health Service Employers Agency, nursing and other appropriate organisations to establish standard criteria in relation to the entry requirements, education qualifications and training for care assistants across the health service.***

Summary of Recommendations in Chapter Four

The Commission recommends that the nursing profession take greater responsibility for the regulation and practice of the profession and for ensuring professional leadership in nursing and midwifery. (4.2)

The Commission recommends that the profession take greater control over its own destiny through ownership of An Bord Altranais (the Board). (4.12)

The Commission recommends that section 6(1) of the 1985 Act be amended to provide that the general concern of the Board shall be the protection of the public through the promotion of high standards of professional education, training and practice and professional conduct among nurses and midwives. (4.13)

The Commission recommends that section 51(2) of the 1985 Act be amended to provide that it shall be a function of the Board to give professional guidance and support on matters relating to clinical practice as well as giving guidance on all matters relating to ethical conduct and behaviour. (4.14)

The Commission recommends that the Board, as a matter of urgency, review the guidelines in relation to the administration or application of non-prescribed drugs by nurses and midwives. (4.15)

The Commission recommends that the 1985 Act be amended to provide that the Board shall consist of a maximum of twenty-eight members appointed in the following way:

(a) eight nurses resident in the State, three of whom are representative of nurses engaged in clinical practice in general nursing (one of whom shall be working in care of the elderly), two of whom are representative of nurses engaged in clinical practice in psychiatric nursing and three of whom are nurses engaged in clinical practice in each of the following disciplines, sick children's, mental handicap and public health nursing, respectively, elected by nurses;

(b) five nurses resident in the State who are engaged in nursing education in each of the following disciplines, general, sick children's, psychiatric, mental handicap and public health, respectively, elected by nurses;

(c) five nurses resident in the State who are engaged in nursing management in each of the following disciplines, general, sick children's, psychiatric, mental handicap and public health, respectively, elected by nurses;

(d) three midwives resident in the State, one of whom is engaged in midwifery education, one of whom is engaged in midwifery management and one of whom is engaged in clinical practice, elected by midwives;

(e) three persons appointed by the Minister, representative of the interests of the general public, who are not nurses or former nurses; and

(f) not more than four persons (other than candidates unsuccessful in elections to the Board) nominated by the Board at its discretion and appointed by the Minister, representative of any areas of the health services or of nursing education or of a category of nursing not elected to the Board. (4.21)

The Commission recommends that the 1985 Act be amended to provide that the term of office for members of the Board be of six years duration with half the number going out of office every three years. (4.22)

The Commission recommends that section 10 of the 1985 Act be amended to provide a new sub-section providing that the appointment of members to the Board by the Minister shall be made within eight weeks of notice to him of the necessity to make such appointments. (4.23)

The Commission recommends that the Board:

- profile all candidates in the Board's newsletter with a view to affording each candidate an equal opportunity;

- provide a free copy of the register for all candidates;

- investigate how to encourage nurses and midwives to run as candidates;

- continue to allow nurses and midwives attend meetings of the board, so that they would become familiar with the work of the Board; and

- simplify the voting system (this might include "Freepost" return of ballot paper and the provision of swipe cards (complete with PIN number) to facilitate completion of the ballot paper). (4.25)

The Commission recommends that the Board consider the more active use of section 13 of the 1985 Act (which provides for the establishment of committees by the Board) to broaden even further the range of expertise available to it in considering issues of concern to the profession. (4.26)

The Commission recommends that the 1985 Act be amended to provide for the following revised fitness to practise procedures. The revised framework provides for the setting up of three ad hoc sub-committees drawn from the membership of the Fitness to Practise Committee. A person should not be a member of more than one sub-committee dealing with the same complaint(s) under the revised fitness to practise procedures. (4.32)

The Commission recommends that there should be an ad hoc preliminary screening sub-committee, composed of three members of the Fitness to Practise Committee. (4.33)

If a complaint relates to a health issue, the Commission recommends that there should be an ad hoc health sub-committee, composed of five members of the Fitness to Practise Committee (one of whom must be a representative of the public interest) to investigate the issue. (4.34)

If a complaint relates to a misconduct issue, the Commission recommends that there should be an ad hoc professional conduct sub-committee, composed of five members of the Fitness to Practise Committee (one of whom must be a representative of the public interest and one of whom must be of the same discipline as the nurse) to investigate the issue. (4.35)

The Commission recommends that section 42(1) of the 1985 Act be amended to extend the full range of sanctions to cases of conviction for an indictable offence. (4.38)

The Commission recommends that the 1985 Act be amended to allow for a sanction to be imposed by agreement between the nurse or midwife and the Board. (4.39)

The Commission recommends that section 39 of the 1985 Act be amended to allow a nurse or midwife twenty-one days from the date of service of notification of a decision to apply to the High Court for cancellation of such a decision. The revised time period should also apply in relation to an application to the High Court by the Board for confirmation of a sanction. (4.41)

The Commission recommends that the 1985 Act be amended to remove the requirement of application to the High Court where the Board and nurse or midwife have reached agreement on the sanction to be imposed. (4.42)

The Commission recommends that any sanction, other than a sanction pursuant to section 41 of the 1985 Act (which allows the Board to advise, admonish or censure a nurse) imposed against a person under the fitness to practise procedures, should be entered forthwith on the register against the name of the person for the duration of the sanction. The register should be open to inspection by members of the public. (4.43)

The Commission acknowledges the request from midwives for recognition of their distinct identity and recommends that the title of the amending legislation should be the Nurses and Midwives Act. (4.44)

The Commission recommends the 1985 Act be amended to provide for the restoration of a separate statutory midwives committee consisting of eight members. It is recommended that such a committee consist of the three elected midwife members of the Board and five registered midwives appointed by the Board. In light of the increasing demand for domiciliary midwifery services, it is recommended that one of the five registered midwives appointed by the Board should be a midwife currently engaged in providing domiciliary midwifery services. This committee should have power to draft the scope of practice for midwives subject to approval of the Board. In the case of an allegation of professional misconduct against a midwife, four of the midwives committee plus one member of the Fitness to Practise Committee, representative of the interests of the general public, should be constituted by the Chair of the Fitness to Practise Committee as a professional conduct sub-committee reporting back to the Board with recommendations. At least one of the midwives on the professional conduct sub-committee should be an elected member of the Board. Health cases can be heard by a health sub-committee appointed in the normal way by the Chair of the Fitness to Practise Committee. (4.45)

The Commission recommends that the 1985 Act be amended to provide that a nurse or midwife may apply to have her or his name removed from the register as is provided in section 33 of the Medical Practitioners Act 1978. (4.46)

The Commission recommends that sub-paragraph (b) of section 39(1) of the 1985 Act be deleted (thus removing non-payment of the retention fee from the fitness to practise procedure) and that part III of the 1985 Act (dealing with registration) be amended to provide that after notice is given to the address on the register, the names of nurses who fail to pay the annual retention fee within the time provided by the rules, may be deleted from the register at any meeting of the Board after such time has expired. Notice of such a deletion is sent to the nurse or midwife involved, and the name can be restored to the register on application, on payment of a penalty fee. The rules should provide that the period within which the retention fee must be paid is from 1st January to 30th April in each year. (4.49)

The Commission recommends that the 1985 Act be amended to entitle the Board to require any nurse or midwife to satisfy it as to her or his relevant competencies, failing which the Board could require an up-date on skills and knowledge, as a condition of retention of name on the register, provided the purpose would be for the protection of the public even in the absence of any complaint. Rules for the exercise of this power, which are fair and equitable, would have to be drawn up by the Board and monitored to ensure that the concerns expressed about its exercise would not be realised. (4.51)

The Commission recommends the Board keep the criteria for recording of post-registration qualifications under constant review. (4.52)

The Commission recommends that the rules of the Board should be amended to provide that on payment of the retention fee each year, every nurse and midwife should be obliged to give particulars of the names of the employer and the position held as of 1st January in each year, such information to appear on the register. (4.53)

The Commission recommends that section 30 of the 1985 Act (which allows for registration with the Board of persons in a profession ancillary to nursing) be deleted. The Commission also recommends that the Minister establish a working party comprised of the Department of Health and Children, the Health Service Employers Agency, nursing and other appropriate organisations, to establish standard criteria in relation to the entry requirements, education qualifications and training for care assistants across the health service. (4.55)

Preparation for the Profession

5.1   This chapter outlines concerns in relation to the current framework for the pre-registration education of nurses. The Commission, in considering the issue was conscious of the need to ensure that nurses are equipped to meet the rapidly changing and complex demands of the health service into the next century. The Commission recommends a revised framework for the pre-registration education of nurses, together with a strategic plan for the future direction of nurse educators.

The Traditional or Apprenticeship Model of Training

5.2   The traditional model of pre-registration training and education for nurses has been described as an "apprenticeship" model. This system, regardless of discipline, was based on classroom instruction and practical training, predominantly in a hospital setting. The arrangement of student nurse training consisted of a student working on a ward and attending lectures. It was mainly characterised by a hospital-based training pattern where the student was an employee and part of the staffing complement of a hospital. The examination and assessment system consisted of continuous assessment of clinical skills through a proficiency assessment format and a final written examination conducted by An Bord Altranais (the Board).

5.3   Formerly, a student seeking to become a nurse could enter one of four nursing pre-registration programmes - general, psychiatric, sick children's and mental handicap nursing. After successful completion of one programme and registration, a further eighteen month programme could be undertaken in order to register in another of these four disciplines of nursing. However, following the EU Directive 89/595/EEC, availability of such shorter courses became limited. A recent change to these education pathways was the requirement of registration as a general, psychiatric or mental handicap nurse in order to pursue an education programme in sick children's nursing. Following registration and experience in one of these four disciplines of nursing, a nurse can pursue an education programme to seek registration as a nurse tutor. Registration as a general nurse is required to pursue an education programme in midwifery and registration as a midwife is required to pursue an education programme in public health nursing.

5.4   The Board, under the Nurses Act 1985, is charged with the responsibility for the control of nurse education. The system operates and is controlled under the Nurses Rules 1988 (as amended) and criteria for the implementation of the syllabi of training. The Board's criteria, which must fulfil the European Union Directives on general nursing and midwifery, provide guidance to schools of nursing on the implementation of their programme of nurse education and training. There are currently no EU Directives on sick children's, mental handicap and psychiatric nursing. Individual schools of nursing are monitored through an inspection system by the Board, such an inspection being carried out at least once every five years in accordance with the Nurses Rules 1988 (as amended).

The Transition to a Diploma Programme

5.5   The apprenticeship model was evaluated by the Board and a number of weaknesses were identified which militated against a beneficial experience for the student nurse. These included a lack of preparation for certain duties, a lack of clinical teaching, an emphasis on work rather than learning and an involvement in non-nursing duties. In the light of this evaluation, the traditional apprenticeship model of pre-registration nurse training and education has been replaced by a new registration/diploma-based programme in general, psychiatric and mental handicap nursing. The diploma-based pre-registration education programme is offered by schools of nursing in association with colleges/universities. The objective of the transition to the new programme was to enhance nursing education and training. This was in line with key recommendations contained in the report *The Future of Nurse Education and Training in Ireland* published by the Board in 1994.

5.6   The first nursing registration/diploma programme, following approval by the Board, commenced on a pilot basis in University College Hospital, Galway, in association with the National University of Ireland - Galway, in October, 1994. The programme of education commenced in University College Hospital Galway became known as the "Galway Model". The programme was extended to four schools of nursing in 1995 and was further extended to nine additional schools of nursing in 1996 and to thirteen additional schools of nursing in 1997. The remaining schools of nursing, of which there are a small number in mental handicap and psychiatry, completed the transition to the registration/diploma programme in 1998.

Main Features of the Diploma Programme

5.7   The main features of the registration/diploma programme have been described as follows:

- applicants are selected for places in schools of nursing offering the programme through the national Nursing Applications Centre (see paragraph 5.32);

- students on the programme register with the associated university/college as well as on the candidate register of the Board and have limited access to the facilities of the university/college;

- the associated university/college validates the curriculum and provides up to 500 lecture hours in the areas of biological and social sciences to the first year students;

- students are examined and assessed by the associated university/college throughout the programme, in addition to undergoing the examination and assessment procedures prescribed in the Rules of the Board;

- the third-level fees are funded by the Department of Health and Children and paid through the relevant health board/hospital/agency;

- students on the programme are supernumerary to service requirements and are not therefore paid a salary;

- the existing "traditional" student nurses' service is replaced by an appropriate grade/skill mix of registered nurses and other grades;

- students receive a maintenance grant of £3,000 per annum paid in monthly instalments;

- principal textbooks up to a value of £200 are supplied to students without charge by the participating schools of nursing at the commencement of the programme;

- students are also supplied with uniforms purchased for them by the health board/hospital/agency;

- students are provided with free meals in designated hospitals on a seven day per week basis; and

- students are responsible for arranging their own accommodation and an accommodation officer is available to assist and advise them after offers of places on the programme have been accepted.

5.8   The registration/diploma programme conforms to the syllabus and Rules of the Board and relevant EU Directives. The arrangements that have been put in place between the schools of nursing and the university/college participating in the programme involve the schools of nursing remaining as distinct entities within the health service. Generally, the Matron/Director of Nursing retains overall responsibility for the school of nursing which is managed by a Principal Nurse Tutor. The associated universities/colleges have each established a department/centre of nursing studies which is a distinct entity within the institute. This department/centre of nursing studies is managed by a nurse with appropriate academic qualifications and experience.

5.9   The programme is of 156 weeks duration (three consecutive years) and meets the 4,600 hours of theoretical and clinical instruction required by the Rules of the Board and specified in the terms of EU Directive 89/595/EEC. The theory content of the programme (including study time) is of fifty-eight weeks duration. A total of eighty-six weeks is allocated to clinical placements (nursing practice). Clinical placement co-ordinators have been appointed in each training hospital/agency to advise, encourage and facilitate students to achieve the maximum benefit from clinical placements. Nursing practice development co-ordinators have also been appointed to help ensure the optimum learning environment for student nurses on clinical placement, in addition to other nursing practice functions.

Issues Raised During the Consultative Process

5.10   The introduction of the registration/diploma programme was widely welcomed as offering new educational opportunities for the nursing profession. It was seen as beginning the process of placing the education of nurses on a par with that of other professions in the health service. The registration/diploma programme was also seen as possibly leading to a more broadly educated, more analytical and self-confident profession, whilst retaining the core value of caring for patients.

5.11   However, numerous concerns were expressed to the Commission in relation to the current model of the registration/diploma programme, both by those attending the consultative fora organised by the Commission and in written submissions. These related primarily to the lack of consultation and perceived lack of planning in relation to the extension of the "Galway Model" registration/diploma programme to other schools of nursing and third-level institutes. The strict requirements in relation to the content of the programme were also seen as creating difficulties. Third-level institutes are required to teach all of the biological/social science subjects in the first year of the programme. This requirement, together with the amount of nursing theory and practice taught by schools of nursing, was seen as placing excessive demands on students.

Evaluation of the Diploma Programme

5.12   In April, 1996 a comprehensive independent external evaluation of the "Galway Model" registration/diploma programme commenced. This is being undertaken by Professor Helen Simons and a team from the School of Education and the School of Nursing, University of Southampton. The evaluation is primarily a case study of the general nursing registration/diploma programme in the pilot site of Galway. A comprehensive evaluation of the registration/diploma programme for psychiatric nursing was not part of the brief. The psychiatric nursing programme, for which there was a single intake of twelve students in October 1995, is considered in the context of the Galway case study. The overall aim of the evaluation is to examine the effectiveness of the "pilot" programme in practice in the Galway site and to ascertain whether the significant issues identified in this site are similar to those arising in the additional sites which commenced in October 1995. This exercise is due to be completed shortly. In light of the detailed evaluation being carried out by Professor Simons and the evaluation team, the Commission did not examine in detail the issues relating to the provision of the registration/diploma programme.

5

5.13   The Commission understands that these issues are dealt with in the external evaluation report. The Commission recommends that immediate action is taken by the Board in the light of this report. The Board should ensure that the concerns of the registration/diploma students and nurse educators are addressed as a matter of urgency so that changes can be implemented by third-level institutes and schools of nursing by October 1999 at the latest.

Concerns in Relation to a Diploma Model of Education

5.14   Apart from the issues in relation to course content and implementation of the registration/ diploma programme, there were concerns relating to the concept of the diploma programme. The programme was seen by many as half way between the traditional apprenticeship model of education and a degree programme. There appears to be a concern that the registration/diploma programme, even if issues of course content are resolved, will not offer nursing students the full educational and personal benefits of a third-level education. Students under the programme are not seen as "real" third-level students and neither are they traditional apprentice students. The students have not been incorporated into the third-level student body. The schools of nursing under the registration/diploma programme still provide a substantial proportion of the theoretical and clinical education to student nurses. It was suggested that much of the education was still largely didactic and did not reflect the culture of self-directed learning in third-level education. It was also suggested that the programme did not reflect international trends in nursing education. Students nurses in Australia, New Zealand, Canada and the United States of America are educated to degree level. In Northern Ireland the pre-registration education of student nurses recently came under the aegis of Queens University, Belfast.

International Developments in Pre-Registration Nursing Education

5.15   The Commission engaged Mark Tyrrell to undertake a literature review on international developments in nursing education. The review identified the increasing integration of pre-registration nursing education into the third-level sector. Student nurses in Australia and the United States of America have had third-level college-based pre-registration degree programmes for a number of years. In Canada, all schools of nursing are currently working towards a baccalaureate degree as the sole entry criterion for nursing by the year 2000 (AARN, 1989). In the United Kingdom students are educated to diploma level under Project 2000 which commenced in the 1980's. Four year pre-registration degree programmes have also been available for many years in the United Kingdom. Since 1997 pre-registration nursing education in Northern Ireland is the responsibility of Queens University. There have been calls in recent years from nursing leaders and the Royal College of Nursing in the United Kingdom for pre-registration nursing education to move from diploma to degree level.

The Transition to Pre-Registration Degree Programmes in Other Countries

5.16   In the literature review undertaken by Mark Tyrrell, the rationale for integrating pre-registration nursing education into the third-level sector at degree level was identified as the need to prepare nurses better for an ever more complex and technological system of health provision (Hart, 1985). There appeared to be a strong view that the nurse of the future required greater theoretical underpinning of her traditional clinical skills. Graduate education was viewed as offering nurses a more effective base on which to develop their practice skills and master a wide variety of skills. It was argued that the combination of sound formal education and reflective practice in a collegial atmosphere was most likely to produce expert practitioners. As stated previously there have been many calls for pre-registration nursing education in the United Kingdom to move from a diploma to a degree programme. The Royal College of Nursing (RCN) has proposed a degree programme for pre-registration nursing education (RCN, 1997). The RCN concluded that the Project 2000 diploma programme was developed to meet health care needs in the year 2000. However, they were of the view that the proposed degree programme would go further in equipping the competent professional practitioner with the necessary skills to integrate nursing practice with other health care workers to meet the health care needs in a rapidly changing world. Others have put forward similar arguments for the transition to a degree programme, stating that the new expectations for the year 2000 and beyond demand education to equip practitioners not just to be prepared but to be able to be proactive in the practice of health care (Clarke and Warr, 1995).

5.17   On a cautionary note the clinical skills of nurses graduating from some degree programmes appear to have been a cause of concern to health service employers in Australia (University of Newcastle et al, 1997). However, it was identified that after one year of nursing practice, graduates demonstrated an improvement in their ability to prioritise work, manage the delivery of care and in their technical skills (Robertson, 1993).

A Degree Programme versus a Diploma Programme

5.18   The Commission considered at length the future pre-registration education requirements of nurses. It was conscious of the increasing complexity and pace of technological development in the health services. The nurse of the future will be required to possess increased flexibility and the ability to work autonomously. Internationally, graduate education is being increasingly demanded of the nurse of the future. The Commission was also conscious that the health service of the future will require greater inter-disciplinary co-operation in the delivery of health care. All other professionals in the acute health care service have graduate status and if inter-disciplinary health care teams are to function effectively, all participants should have equality of status.

5.19   The Commission considered that nursing students should be educated to degree level and be fully integrated within the third-level education sector. A degree programme will provide nurses with a level of theoretical underpinning which will allow them develop their clinical skills to a greater extent and to respond to future challenges in health care. The Commission considered that there are great benefits to nurses and nursing by their integration within the educational and research culture of third-level institutes. Such integration will allow nurses to develop and examine their practice to a much greater extent than heretofore. **The Commission therefore, recommends that the Minister for Health and Children (the Minister) facilitate the transition of pre-registration nursing education into third-level institutes at degree level.**

Professional Status of Registered Nurses

5.20   The Commission in recommending the move to pre-registration nursing education to a degree programme does not consider that the development will impact on the professional status of existing registered nurses. Internationally the experience has been that developments in the pre-registration education of nurses have not impacted on the professional status or career prospects of existing registered nurses. This reflects the experience of other professional groupings such as accountancy where there have been developments in the educational preparation for entry to the profession. However, the Commission considers that health service providers need to be more flexible and creative in considering applications for support and funding from existing registered nurses and midwives wishing to avail of the increasing range of educational opportunities, which had not been available to them on registration (see chapter six of the report).

A Generic Model of Education

5.21   In the transition to pre-registration education degree programmes, there has been a debate in many countries on the model of education programme. Pre-registration nursing degree programmes in Australia follow a generic model whereby at the end of the programme, students are qualified to work in a variety of settings such as general nursing, psychiatric nursing, children's nursing and community nursing. Midwifery is not included in the generic programme. However, there are concerns in relation to the generic model of pre-registration nursing education, particularly in relation to psychiatric nursing where a student could graduate and enter practice as a generic nurse with little or no theoretical and/or clinical experience of the discipline. The Commission considered a generic model of pre-registration nursing education, but ultimately was of the view that there was a need to retain distinct pre-registration education programmes for general, mental handicap and psychiatric nursing. The Commission was of the view that there was a need to retain the distinct identity of the three disciplines to ensure the competence of nurses to work in these areas on registration, particularly in the areas of mental handicap and mental health. The Commission was of the view that retaining the distinct identity of mental handicap and psychiatric nursing was essential, in order to continue to attract student nurses to these crucial areas of the health service.

A Pre-Registration Degree Programme in Nursing

5.22   ***The Commission recommends that the future framework for the pre-registration education of nurses be based on a four year degree programme in each of the disciplines of general, psychiatric and mental handicap nursing, approved by the Board, which will encompass clinical placements, including twelve months continuous clinical placement as a paid employee of the health service.*** The Commission considers it essential that nursing education continues to have a strong clinical foundation. The granting of a degree will entitle the holder to registration with the Board. The academic year should be based around the existing academic calendars for third-level institutes. Nursing students should be integrated with the general third-level student body to facilitate exposure to a greater range of disciplines and ideas outside of the health services. Focused clinical placements to ensure that learning is applied, would take place over the initial two or three year period but would be largely fitted into the academic calendar. Nursing students would be supernumerary for these initial placements. Nursing students holiday entitlement would be broadly in line with existing third-level students on other courses. Nursing students would not be supernumerary during the twelve months continuous clinical placement.

5.23   The Commission considers that an important component of the programme would be twelve months continuous clinical placement as paid health service employees. Such placement is considered essential in ensuring the clinical competence of nurses on graduation and registration. Candidates should be assessed for clinical competence during the course of the year by third-level institutes under a system approved by the Board. It is envisaged that the twelve months continuous clinical placement would take place between the third and fourth year of the programme. Normal student holiday entitlement would not apply for the duration of the twelve months clinical placement. Consideration should be given to the placement of students in appropriate clinical settings in smaller hospitals, in addition to placement in the main teaching hospitals. These placements might take place as part of the twelve months continuous clinical placement. Students during this period would be entitled to holidays on the same basis as staff nurses. Following completion of the twelve months continuous clinical placement students would return to the third-level institutes for a period to apply theoretical knowledge to their clinical experience. On completion of the course, a third-level examination would take place and successful candidates would be awarded a degree, which could be an honours degree. The award of a degree would entitle a nurse to be registered with the Board.

5.24   The academic element of the nursing degree programmes should be based on curricula with distinct courses (modules or units) with associated credit weightings. This would allow students whose primary degree is in general nursing to apply for a degree in psychiatric or mental handicap nursing and to be given credit for existing courses covered in a general nursing degree and relevant to psychiatric or mental handicap nursing (or vice versa). This approach of awarding academic credits should ensure that a person having spent four years obtaining a general nursing degree would not have to spend a further three years obtaining a psychiatric or mental handicap nursing degree. This approach would also mean that nursing students may transfer credits to other third-level courses.

5.25   The Commission recognises that the proposal of a third-level institute-based degree programme will need to be carefully implemented. It is essential that there be a carefully planned period to allow for transition to the new degree programme. Career guidance counsellors would need to be advised of the changes well in advance. Third-level institutes, schools of nursing and health service providers would need to prepare for the introduction of the new programme which should be introduced in a carefully planned manner. The existing linkages between teaching hospitals and third-level institutes need to be further developed.

5.26   ***The Commission recommends that a forum be established by the Minister involving the third-level institutes, schools of nursing, health service providers and the Board. The objective of the forum should be to agree a strategy for the implementation of degree level pre-registration education and it should be funded by the State.*** Such a forum should also address the anomalies arising from the transition to the graduate programme and strengthen links amongst all involved in pre-registration nurse education. The report of Professor Simons and her team following the evaluation of the "Galway Model" registration/diploma programme and the lessons learned from the transition to the diploma programme should inform the forum in its deliberations on the development of a degree programme. ***The Commission recommends that the Minister, following consultation with the Minister for Education, Science and Technology, appoint an independent chair of the forum. In addition, the Commission recommends that the forum report within two years of its establishment.***

5.27   Health service providers, schools of nursing and third-level institutes should work together to draw up curricula for validation by the third-level institutes and accreditation by the Board.

Transition to the Pre-Registration Degree Programme

5.28   There was much criticism of the phased introduction of the registration/diploma nursing programme during the consultative process undertaken by the Commission. There was criticism of the decision to extend the "Galway model" registration/diploma programme prior to its full evaluation and in the absence of consultation with nurse tutors, other educationalists and the third-level institutes. The resultant rush to commence the pre-registration diploma in other third-level institutes, once it had commenced in the National University of Ireland - Galway, resulted in students, third-level institutes and nurse educators encountering greater difficulties than otherwise might have been expected in the transition to the registration/diploma programme.

5.29   In order to ensure a planned and effective transition to the third-level institute-based degree programme, the Commission is strongly of the opinion that a date should be set at the outset for the commencement of the degree programme. ***The Commission recommends that all third-level institutes and disciplines of nursing should commence the pre-registration degree programme on a specified date.*** This would give the third-level institutes, nurse educators and health service providers time to prepare for the transition. An essential element would be time to allow nurse educators prepare personally for a possible transfer into third-level institutes by upgrading their academic qualifications, if necessary. It would also allow time for the development of curricula in detailed discussions between third-level institutes, health service providers and the Board. No third-level institute or discipline should commence the programme prior to the agreed date. If any third-level institute or discipline commenced prior to the agreed date it would probably result in demands from all the other groups involved in pre-registration nursing education to commence the programme and would result in a recurrence of many of the difficulties encountered in the transition to the registration/diploma programme.

5.30 **The Commission**, having considered the need for nurse educators, third-level institutes and career guidance counsellors to prepare adequately for the transition to the pre-registration degree programme, **recommends that the start of the academic year in 2002 be specified as the commencement date of the degree programme.** The date of the start of the academic year in 2002 would allow two years for the forum of interested parties on pre-registration education to report, followed by a two year period for students making their Leaving Certificate subject choices. This would allow students wishing to do nursing to adjust their Leaving Certificate subject selection to take account of any revised selection criteria. The first intake of students into the degree programme would be those completing their Leaving Certificate in 2002. It is stressed that no third-level institute or health service provider should commence the degree programme prior to that date.

Accreditation by the Board

5.31 The role of the Board remains central to pre-registration education. In future the Board would ensure the desired outcomes by accrediting:

- the content of the degrees offered by third-level institutes (the Board could set up sub-committees to discuss and approve each programme as it is submitted to them);

- clinical areas used for the placement of students;

- and the system of assessment for clinical placements throughout the programme and, in particular, during the twelve months continuous clinical placement.

In achieving this, the Board would work closely with Departments of Nursing in third-level institutes and health service providers. The Commission does not see the necessity for the Board to register students during their education at third-level institutes. However, the Board should consider registering students during their twelve months clinical placement.

The Administration of the Selection and Recruitment of Student Nurses

5.32 In 1995 the Minister established a Nursing Applications Centre on a pilot basis to provide a national centralised application and selection system for applicants seeking places on the new pre-registration nursing registration/diploma programme. The Nursing Applications Centre has managed three annual intakes to the programme. The Department of Health and Children engaged Price Waterhouse management consultants to carry out an evaluation of the Nursing Applications Centre in 1997. Price Waterhouse also acted as project managers for the application/selection process for the 1997 student intake as part of their evaluation of the current procedures. This arrangement was intended to facilitate the introduction, on an experimental basis, of certain modifications to the procedures employed in previous years with the objective of streamlining the application/selection process. Price Waterhouse reported a number of difficulties in the operation of the selection system for student nurses (Department of Health, 1997).

5.33   The Commission is of the view that the management of applications from a large number of candidates requires particular expertise if it is to operate in an administratively efficient manner. The increasing range of educational opportunities available to candidates also needs to be considered in ensuring the administrative efficiency of any selection process. The Commission met with the Central Applications Office (CAO) to discuss its operation. The CAO has operated successfully for a number of years in the selection of candidates for third-level institutes. In discussions with the CAO it appears that the selection of nursing students could be successfully incorporated within the existing CAO system. The incorporation of nursing into the CAO system would also allow for a cross referencing between candidates who have applied for other courses in the CAO system and nursing.

5.34   *The Commission recommends that the CAO administer the application system for pre-registration nursing education.* The current CAO application form allows candidates to indicate their order of preference for degree and diploma courses. In discussions with the CAO, it was suggested that the current CAO system could readily accommodate a third range of options under the heading of nursing. This would allow candidates for nursing to indicate their order of preference for the third-level institute in which they wish to undertake a nursing degree. The three disciplines of pre-registration nursing (general, psychiatric and mental handicap) could be differentiated within the CAO system. Candidates applying for nursing would apply for a degree in a discipline of nursing at a third-level institute in their order of preference. The allocation of students for clinical placements would be managed by the third-level institutes.

5.35   The system could also encompass applications for particular schools of nursing under the current diploma programme prior to the implementation of a third-level institute-based degree programme. *The Commission recommends that the administration of the pre-registration nursing application system for the current diploma programmes be transferred to the CAO, in advance of the move to a third-level institute-based degree qualification.*

Selection Criteria

5.36   *The Commission recommends that admission to nursing be on the basis of the attainment of a specified Leaving Certificate standard plus an interview.* In extensive consultations with the profession, the predominant view was that the interview be retained. The specified Leaving Certificate standard could be set as the matriculation requirement of each individual third-level institute, provided it met entry requirements set by the Board. It is important that nursing students should be admitted to third-level institutes with the option of transferring to other courses. Candidates would be placed in order of merit on the basis of a combination of points from their Leaving Certificate results and an interview. The ratio of points to be awarded between the Leaving Certificate results and interview could be determined initially by the forum. In discussions with the CAO, the Commission was informed that the CAO system will not readily incorporate an interview after Leaving Certificate results. If an interview takes place following the Leaving Certificate results a candidate will not receive a first round offer for nursing from the CAO. This could operate to the disadvantage of nursing in competing for high calibre candidates. It has been the experience of the CAO that candidates accept the first offer they have been made, even if it might not have been their first choice. This is particularly the case if there is a long time lag between the first round offer and a subsequent offer. Interviews should therefore be conducted prior to the Leaving Certificate results and organised on a regional basis by a central organising body (this function is currently carried out by the Local Appointments Commission) to ensure consistency and administrative efficiency.

5.37   The Commission considered the use of an assessment or biodata test as an aid to determining the suitability of candidates for nursing. There was much criticism of the use of an assessment test in the selection of student nurses in 1997. However, the Commission has been informed that there has been further development of the assessment or biodata test in 1998. Experience to date indicates that the test can be a useful objective measure of suitability for all disciplines of nursing. The same scoring grid is not used in relation to each of the disciplines and the test can serve as an objective measure of the characteristics sought in candidates for each discipline.

5.38   *The Commission recommends that the following selection system be used for each discipline of nursing under the proposed degree programme:*

General Nursing

General nursing has the largest number of candidates for nursing. The Nursing Application Centre received 3,948 applications in 1998, for 734 places. Application would be made in the normal way to the CAO by February each year. The Commission does not consider it efficient or effective to interview all the candidates applying for general nursing, if the number of applicants continues at current levels. Therefore *the Commission recommends that the biodata test or other suitable assessment test should continue to be used as a mechanism of assessing the suitability of candidates for interview in general nursing and also as an aid for the interviewers in assessing suitability. The Commission also recommends that there is on-going validation of the assessment or biodata test and its usefulness.* The results of the interviews would be forwarded to the CAO and combined with Leaving Certificate results to place candidates in order of merit. In summary:

*   candidates apply to the CAO for general nursing indicating their preferred third-level institutes (the school of nursing would not be indicated);

*   all candidates sit the assessment or biodata test;

*   the numbers to be interviewed to be determined according to the results;

*   chosen candidates interviewed through a central organising body (to be held in regional centres);

*   the interviewers to use the results of the biodata test as an aid in the interview process;

*   results of interviews given to CAO; and

*   places offered on the basis of leaving certificate results combined with interview marks, the proportion to be determined initially by the forum.

Psychiatric and Mental Handicap Nursing

The number of candidates applying for psychiatric and mental handicap nursing is much smaller than for general nursing. In 1998, there were 968 applications for psychiatric nursing for 201 places and 550 applications for mental handicap nursing for 173 places. *The Commission considers that the assessment or biodata test would be a useful aid to those involved in interviewing candidates for psychiatric and mental handicap nursing and therefore recommends its continued use in the selection of candidates for these disciplines.* Regional interviews could be organised through a central organising body composed of panels of suitably experienced psychiatric or mental handicap nurses. Separate interview boards would operate for each discipline. In summary:

*   candidates apply to the CAO for psychiatric and/or mental handicap nursing indicating their preferred third-level institutes (the school of nursing would not be indicated);

- all candidates sit the assessment or biodata test;

- interview through a central organising body (to be held in regional centres);

- the interviewers to use the results of the biodata test as an aid in the interview process;

- results of interviews given to CAO; and

- places offered on a combination of leaving certificate results and interview marks, the proportion to be determined initially by the forum.

The Adelaide Hospital Society

5.39   **The Commission recommends that the Adelaide Hospital Society continues to have a special relationship with the Faculty of Health Sciences in Trinity College Dublin in the recruitment of students for the degree programme.** The Commission envisages that such recruitment takes place outside the CAO system until such time as the society and the CAO have agreed a mutually acceptable method of student recruitment.

The Interview Process

5.40   **The Commission recommends that interview procedures are carefully formulated to obtain universal standards within each discipline whilst allowing interviewers determine the vocational commitment and suitability of applicants.**

The Role of the Board in the Interview Process

5.41   **The Commission recommends that the Board have the responsibility of overseeing the interview process in the selection of candidates for the degree programme.** It is envisaged that the Board will contract out the organisation of the interviews to a central organising body. **The Commission recommends that the Board keep the systems used in the selection of students for nursing under constant review to ensure the continuing use of best practice. The cost of administering the selection process should be met by the State.**

Funding the Degree Programme

5.42   The Commission considers that the funding of the proposed degree programme should remain under the aegis of the Department of Health and Children during the initial transition period. It is important that the funding of nursing degree programmes is clearly protected during the transition period and that those most familiar with the needs of nursing are responsible for its funding. Once nursing has been integrated into the third-level institutes, the funding of pre-registration nursing education should become the responsibility of the Department of Education, Science and Technology in two stages. In the first stage, the funding for nursing should be red-circled within the funding to the Department of Education, Science and Technology. When the degree programme is well established, the funding could be integrated within the general third-level education budgets. It is envisaged that the degree programme will operate in the same manner as all other degree programmes within the third-level education sector under the remit of the free education system. Under such a system, the State pays the course fees provided a student does not have a previous degree from an Irish third-level institute. The Commission is conscious that the integration of nursing students onto the campuses of third-level institutes may require substantial capital investment.

The Nursing Student Grant System

5.43   The Commission has recommended that pre-registration nursing education becomes incorporated into the third-level education sector, with education modules being organised, which take place around academic semesters. This would allow nursing students to become more like other third-level students with similar holiday periods. Therefore, it is considered by the Commission that the current non-means tested grant of £3,000 to nursing students may no longer be tenable in such a scenario. *Therefore the Commission recommends that the student nursing grant and any student benefits should be the same as those available to other third-level students and be means tested.* The funding formerly available for books should be directed at upgrading nursing libraries. However, as it is envisaged that student nurses will have some supernumerary clinical placements during the initial academic phase of the programme, expenses incurred for travel and accommodation off site should be reimbursed. Students might apply on an individual basis for travel expenses and accommodation costs incurred on clinical placements along the lines of the system used for primary teaching students. Nursing uniforms should continue to be provided, if required.

5.44   *The Commission recommends that the student is paid a salary during the twelve months continuous clinical placement at the level of eighty percent of the first year staff nurse's salary. This is the current level of payment for third year apprenticeship students. The twelve months continuous clinical placement for which a student is paid should also be subsequently reckonable for pension purposes. Following graduation, the Commission recommends that a nurse, who has completed the twelve months continuous clinical placement, should start employment at the second increment point on the staff nurse salary scale.* This will allow a nurse who has completed the four year pre-registration degree programme to start employment on the same salary as graduates of the three year registration/diploma programme, who have completed one year of employment.

Mature Students

5.45   Mature students represent an increasingly important cohort of student nurses. In the United Kingdom, the Royal College of Nursing reported that one third of nursing students were over twenty five years of age and over twenty five percent have dependent children (RCN, 1994). In Ireland twelve percent of those sitting the assessment or biodata test for nursing in 1998 were mature applicants (i.e. over twenty-four years of age). In recognition of the importance of mature applicants for nursing, *the Commission recommends that mature students should have a certain percentage of the third-level places in nursing assigned to them. The Commission recommends the percentage be determined by the third-level institutes in consultation with the Board*. Each third-level institute would determine the selection criteria to be used for mature students in association with a joint interview conducted by health service providers and third-level institutes. The selection process for mature students would operate in parallel with the selection system used for school leavers and should ensure that candidates can cope with the academic rigours of a degree course whilst showing the necessary vocational commitment to nursing.

5.46   The Commission recognises that mature students play an increasingly important role in nursing and midwifery and particularly in psychiatric and mental handicap nursing. Such students bring a particular maturity to the profession and should be encouraged and supported. *The Commission recommends a bursary/sponsorship system be put in place by the Department of Health and Children to promote applications to all disciplines by mature students.* The framework for the operation of the system should be discussed and decided between the Department of Health and Children, service providers and the Board.

The Promotion of the Profession

5.47 Traditionally there has been little difficulty in attracting students to nursing in Ireland. In 1998, there were approximately four applications for each place in nursing. However, this may not always remain the case, particularly if the improved range of employment opportunities continues in the coming years. The range of career options for women in the public and private sector may have a particular impact on the numbers entering nursing. It is hoped that the implementation of the recommendations of the Commission will enhance the attractiveness of the profession. However, the Commission considers that there is a need to promote the profession actively. *The Commission recommends that the Board and the Department of Health and Children examine mechanisms of promoting the profession as a career option among school leavers.*

Improved Gender Balance in the Profession

5.48 Nursing remains a predominantly female profession. Of the total number of nurses and midwives registered at the end of 1996, ninety-three percent were women. It was suggested during the consultative process that certain clinical situations may require a nurse of a particular gender. There was a view that there was a need to improve the gender balance within the profession. It was suggested that there was a need to improve the profile of nursing as a career option amongst males. *The Commission recommends that the Board examine mechanisms of increasing the number of male candidates applying to enter the profession.*

State Enrolled Nurses

5.49 The Commission received a number of submissions from state enrolled nurses regarding their access to conversion courses to become registered nurses. The state enrolled nurse is a United Kingdom qualification which is not recognised in Ireland. During the Depression in the 1930's, registered nurses were regarded as an expensive commodity and individual hospitals began to train assistant nurses to deliver some of the duties of registered nurses at a lesser cost. The government of the United Kingdom reacted to this development by enacting the Nurses Act 1943 with provision for a second-level nurse, the state enrolled nurse, with a two year training programme, lower entry qualifications and whose duties were envisaged as assisting the registered nurse in practical nursing care. The state enrolled nurse qualification came to be regarded as anomalous in the United Kingdom in the 1970's and 1980's. The implementation of Project 2000 on a revised nurse education structure in the United Kingdom resulted in the abolition of training courses for state enrolled nurses and the provision of conversion courses to registered nurse status. The United Kingdom Central Council for Nurses, Midwives and Health Visitors (UKCC) recognises the state enrolled nurse qualification alone as sufficient to access conversion courses. A number of state enrolled nurses who are employed in the Irish health services have asked the Board to assess their qualification and provide appropriate conversion courses in Ireland to allow them the opportunity to convert to registered nurse status in this country.

5.50 There is a conversion course available to state enrolled nurses in Belfast, but it does involve travel to Northern Ireland in order to fulfil clinical placement requirements. Some health boards have facilitated some employees who have a state enrolled nurse qualification to attend these courses. The Commission considered the issue of conversion courses for holders of the state enrolled nurse qualification. The Commission recognises that there is no tradition in Ireland of a registerable nursing qualification other than registered nurse. Similarly, there is no precedent in Ireland for the provision of courses of the type provided for state enrolled nurses in Northern Ireland. Therefore the Commission, having considered the matter, does not recommend any change in the Rules of the Board in relation to the recognition of the state enrolled nurse qualification or the provision of conversion courses in Ireland.

The Role of Nurse Educators

5.51 The Commission, in considering the future direction of pre-registration nursing education, was conscious of the need to develop simultaneously a coherent framework for nurse educators. The high quality and international standing of Irish nurses is due in no small part to the efforts of nurse educators over the years. The Commission recognises the invaluable contribution of nurse tutors to the high international reputation of Irish nurses. The success of any education programme is dependent on the quality and commitment of educators and the future success of the proposed degree programme is primarily dependent on the efforts of nurse educators.

5.52 It is an accepted principle in the public-health service that any restructuring of a service will not result in job losses or a reduction in salary. The Commission supports the application of this principle in the restructuring of pre-registration nursing education. The Commission also recognises that there will be a substantial culture change as a result of the move of pre-registration nursing education into third-level institutes. The Commission agreed that there should be a role for all the existing nurse tutors within the revised educational and health service framework in areas such as the delivery of the pre-registration nursing degree programme, the operation of the twelve months continuous clinical placement and in continuing nursing education.

Northern Ireland

5.53 In Northern Ireland, pre-registration nursing education has moved into Queens University at two campus sites - one in Queens University, Belfast and the other at the Queens Campus in Altnagelvin, Derry. The diploma class for 1997 has already been taken into Queens University and in 1998 all remaining pre-registration students will be moved onto the campus. Although nurse tutors were coming from a third-level education environment, the culture was such that it was difficult to obtain sufficient time to publish articles and carry out research as required for academic appointment. Nurse tutors therefore were transferred to Queens on academic related contracts and specially created posts of nurse lecturer with the same salary as nurse tutors. These posts were specific to the nursing programme. Tutors, with the necessary academic and other qualifications, could compete for academic posts, but there was no automatic entitlement to such posts.

The Academic Career Pathway in the Third Level Sector

5.54 Appointment to a lectureship post is a matter for each third-level institute and appointment is dependent on a prescribed minimum level of academic qualification, together with a background in research and publication. The minimum level of academic qualification may vary from college to college. In one university, the specified minimum academic qualification for appointment as a lecturer was stated to be an honours degree and three years work/study/research experience. However, given the level of competition for such posts, those being appointed often have a much higher level of academic achievement. There is also a variety of contracts for lectureship posts within third-level institutes; some are permanent but other college lecturers are part-time or full-time on a three year roll over contract.

5.55 There is an academic career pathway within the third-level sector. A typical career pathway might be college lecturer, statutory lecturer, associate professor and professorship. There is no automatic entitlement to progression beyond college lecturer. A typical salary for the post of college lecturer is £23,146 to £37,520. The nurse tutor salary scale is £23,090 to £26,000 and the principal nurse tutor salary scale is £24,019 to £28,432. However, Trinity College and University College Cork also operate a bar system within the incremental scale for college lecturer. The bar system means that there is no automatic entitlement to progression beyond a certain point on the salary scale unless the post holder has performed satisfactorily in her/his post. In other universities, there is a grade of assistant lecturer below college lecturer and on a lower salary. If nurse tutors were recruited below the bar into a college lecturer post or at the assistant lecturer level then they would be on a lower salary than their current entitlement. The Commission has already stated that it supports the accepted principle in the public health service that any restructuring of a service will not result in a reduction in salary.

Principal Nurse Tutors

5.56   As stated previously, the high quality and international reputation of Irish nurses is due in no small part to the efforts of nurse educators. The schools of nursing in the teaching hospitals have provided students with a sound educational and vocational foundation. The schools of nursing are seen, by many within the service, as centres of excellence. In each case they are headed by a principal nurse tutor who provides administrative, educational and professional leadership. The unique combination of administrative, educational and professional skills of principal nurse tutors will continue to provide a valuable resource to either third-level institutes or health service providers. Health service providers should discuss with principal nurse tutors, at an early stage, the career options they wish to pursue following the transition to the degree programme. Support should be provided to facilitate the transfer of principal nurse tutors to their chosen career option.

Transition of Nurse Educators to the Third Level Sector

5.57   The Commission recognises that the proposed changes in pre-registration nursing education will have a major impact on the future role of nurse educators. *In recognition of this revised role the Commission recommends that health service employers consult with each nurse tutor currently involved in pre-registration nursing education in relation to her or his desired future career pathway. The purpose of the consultation is to establish whether the tutor wishes to move into third-level education or pursue other avenues in continuing education within the health service or other career options in management or clinical practice. The Commission recommends that health service providers support nurse tutors in upgrading their educational or other qualifications to facilitate their transition to their desired career pathway.*

5.58   Nurse educators who have the appropriate academic qualifications, research activity and history of publication should be afforded the opportunity of competing for posts within the existing academic hierarchy of a third-level institute. *In order to facilitate the transition of as many nurse tutors as possible to the third-level sector, the Commission recommends that those nurse tutors who may not have been successful in competing for academic posts within third-level institutes, or who do not meet the academic and other requirements for appointment as a lecturer within the academic career structure of a third-level institute be appointed as "nurse lecturers" on a personal basis in a similar manner to that developed in Northern Ireland.* These "nurse lecturer" posts would retain the same salary and conditions of nurse tutors. The creation of "nurse lecturer" posts would be a transitional arrangement to cover the initial period of transfer to a university/college-based degree programme. Those appointed to "nurse lecturer" posts should have the possibility of transferring into the academic career pathway at a later stage if they upgraded their academic and other qualifications to the appropriate level.

5.59 ***The Commission recommends that following the transition of pre-registration nursing education to a third-level degree programme, future nurse educators be appointed within the academic career structure of a third-level institute.*** These appointments would be made according to the criteria specified for each post by the individual third-level institutes. Furthermore, the Commission recommends the establishment of a Faculty or Department of Nursing within each third-level institute providing a pre-registration degree programme. These faculties or departments should be comparable with other faculties and departments in third-level institutes. They should be headed by Professors or Deans of Nursing, with an adequate number of lectureships in nursing, to lead and support the programmes.

5.60 ***The Commission recommends that in the transfer to a university/college-based degree programme there should be a number of joint appointments between third-level institutes and health service providers.*** There appears to be no single internationally recognised model for joint appointments from the report prepared for the Commission. However, there is a strong view in countries that have integrated pre-registration nursing education into the third-level sector, that such appointments are essential to the success of the education programmes. These appointments would involve a nurse combining an education role in third-level institutes with a clinical or research role within a health service provider. The detailed arrangements could be determined in discussions between third-level institutes and health service providers. However, prior to the transfer of pre-registration nursing education into third-level institutes, a number of joint appointment posts should be agreed between third-level institutes and the health service providers associated with the pre-registration education programme. Participation of third-level institutes and health service providers in the pre-registration nursing degree programme should be dependent on a number of joint appointments, to be agreed in detailed discussions between the health service provider, the third-level institute, the Board and the Department of Health and Children. The Commission is of the view that serious consideration should be given to joint appointments between third-level institutes and health service providers under the current registration/diploma programme.

Centres of Nursing Education

5.61 Following the transition of the pre-registration nursing degree programme into third-level institutes there will continue to be a need for a strong nursing education presence in the teaching hospitals and health services. Nursing is primarily a practice-based profession and the core of nursing will remain in the delivery of services. ***The Commission recommends that the schools of nursing become centres of nursing education providing a range of educational and training services to nurses in the health services.*** The centres of nursing education would have a crucial role to play during the clinical placement of students on a degree programme. This would be particularly important during the twelve months continuous clinical placement where students are also employees of the health service. The nursing profession as a whole has a responsibility to ensure the high quality of education provided to students preparing for the profession. It is the hallmark of a profession that it takes responsibility for the education of those seeking entry. There will also be a need to support and develop nursing staff in a clinical area to which students are assigned. Staff in these clinical areas need to be aware of the needs of students and to be supported in ensuring that students obtain a beneficial educational outcome from their clinical placement. Such support and development might be delivered through the centres of nursing education.

5.62 In addition to the role of the centres of nursing education during the clinical placement of students on the pre-registration degree programme, there is also a crucial role to be played in the professional development of registered nurses and midwives. The rapidly developing nature of the health services means that it is essential that nurses continuously update their knowledge and skills.

In order to ensure the continuing provision of a high quality nursing service, it is essential that each health service provider supplies a well developed in-service training and educational programme. The Commission envisages nurse tutors with the necessary expertise, who do not wish to transfer to the third-level sector, being employed in this crucial area and overseeing the continuing nursing education programme of health service providers by: identifying the educational needs of nurses; targeting nursing service areas for development; and providing or organising the provision of the continuing educational needs of nurses.

5.63 There will need to be a very close working relationship and liaison between third-level institutes and the teaching hospitals with centres of nursing education. As discussed previously, opportunities for joint appointments between them should be developed. There will be a need to develop both formal and informal links which are strong and clear. The Commission envisages that a framework for such links will be developed in detail during discussions at the forum proposed in paragraph 5.26.

The Commission envisages that the centres of nursing education would have a role in:

- the clinical placement of students during the pre-registration degree programme;

- the post-registration education of nurses;

- the provision of in-service training to nurses; and

- acting as a centre for the professional development of nurses within a health service.

The centres of nursing education would operate under the overall direction of a Director of Nursing or a Chief Nursing Officer. The centres would be staffed by a combination of nurse tutors, clinical placement co-ordinators and practice development co-ordinators.

Clinical Placement Co-ordinators

5.64 Clinical Placement Co-ordinator (CPC) posts were established under the registration/diploma nursing programme. Those in post are skilled clinical nurses and their role is to guide and support student nurses in assigned clinical areas and to ensure that the clinical placements meet the requirements of the education programme with regard to planned experiences and outcomes. CPCs advise, encourage and facilitate students to achieve the maximum outcome from clinical placements. They also ensure that nursing practice assessments are fairly and accurately carried out by the appropriate nurses through effective liaison with nurse tutors, ward and departmental sisters, nursing officers and staff nurses. They play a key role in encouraging the application of theoretical knowledge to nursing practice in the clinical areas. The position of Clinical Placement Co-ordinator is described in a draft job description issued by the Department of Health and Children in 1997 as temporary and experimental and as being at ward sister grade.

5.65 The Commission was conscious of the very positive views expressed by student nurses in relation to the support and encouragement they received from clinical placement co-ordinators in adjusting to and gaining positive learning experiences from their interactions in the clinical environment. The quality of the learning experience from focused clinical placements will be crucial to the success of the pre-registration degree programme. ***The Commission recommends that clinical placement co-ordinators be retained to ensure the quality of clinical placements and the suitability of clinical areas to which students are assigned during clinical placements. The Commission therefore recommends that there be a national evaluation of the role of the clinical placement co-ordinator and the continued development of the post.*** Such posts, which are now at ward sister level, should be permanent and remain responsible to the practice development co-ordinators.

Practice Development Co-ordinators

5.66   Practice Development Co-ordinator posts have developed in hospitals with schools of nursing and some other hospitals in recent years. The posts are at Assistant Director of Nursing level and the main responsibilities are:

(i)   to establish a nursing practice development unit which evaluates, develops, implements and monitors nursing practice in all areas of the hospital;

(ii)   to manage the nursing services quality assurance programmes in such a way as to support and ensure the delivery of the highest standard of patient focused nursing care throughout the hospital; and

(iii)   through supervision of the clinical placement co-ordinators, to ensure that the clinical areas in the hospital, to which student nurses are assigned for clinical placements, provide optimum learning environments and are capable of meeting the learning objectives set by the school of nursing for students.

5.67   ***The Commission recommends that the posts of Practice Development Co-ordinator be given explicit further responsibility to develop clinical nursing research within a health service provider.*** This should include not only the dissemination of information on research, but its implementation and the development of research appreciation skills amongst nurses. The co-ordinator would also oversee, encourage and support the undertaking of research by nurses within a health service provider. In addition to their role of supervising clinical placement co-ordinators, ***the Commission recommends that practice development co-ordinators oversee the organisation of the pre-registration clinical placements. In order to fulfil the proposed combination of educational, management and research functions required in the Practice Development Co-ordinator posts, the Commission recommends that future appointees to the post be educated to masters degree level***. Appropriate clerical and information technology support should be provided to practice development co-ordinators. The practice development co-ordinators would continue to report to the Director of Nursing and would, in future, liaise closely with the Head of a Nursing Department in a third-level institute.

5.68   The Commission envisages that such posts might also be created in areas other than acute teaching hospitals or where there are nursing students. The continuous development of practice in all areas of nursing would have substantial benefits to the quality of patient care. The Commission envisages, for example, the appointment of a practice development co-ordinator for care of the elderly in a health board area.

Summary of Recommendations in Chapter Five

The Commission recommends that the Minister for Health and Children (the Minister) facilitate the transition of pre-registration nursing education into third-level institutes at degree level. (5.19)

The Commission recommends that the future framework for the pre-registration education of nurses be based on a four year degree programme in each of the disciplines of general, psychiatric and mental handicap nursing, approved by the Board, which will encompass clinical placements, including twelve months continuous clinical placement as a paid employee of the health service. (5.22)

The Commission recommends that a forum be established by the Minister involving the third-level institutes, schools of nursing, health service providers and the Board. The objective of the forum should be to agree a strategy for the implementation of degree level pre-registration education and it should be funded by the State. (5.26)

The Commission recommends that the Minister, following consultation with the Minister for Education, Science and Technology, appoint an independent chair of the forum. In addition, the Commission recommends that the forum report within two years of its establishment. (5.26)

The Commission recommends that all third-level institutes and disciplines of nursing should commence the pre-registration degree programme on a specified date. (5.29)

The Commission recommends that the start of the academic year in 2002 be specified as the commencement date of the degree programme. (5.30)

The Commission recommends that the CAO administer the application system for pre-registration nursing education. (5.34)

The Commission recommends that the administration of the pre-registration nursing application system for the current diploma programmes be transferred to the CAO, in advance of the move to a third-level institute-based degree qualification. (5.35)

The Commission recommends that admission to nursing be on the basis of the attainment of a specified Leaving Certificate standard plus an interview. (5.36)

The Commission recommends that the biodata test or other suitable assessment test should continue to be used as a mechanism of assessing the suitability of candidates for interview in general nursing and also as an aid for the interviewers in assessing suitability. (5.38)

The Commission recommends that there is on-going validation of the assessment or biodata test and its usefulness. (5.38)

The Commission considers that the assessment or biodata test would be a useful aid to those involved in interviewing candidates for psychiatric and mental handicap nursing and therefore recommends its continued use in the selection of candidates for these disciplines. (5.38)

The Commission recommends that the Adelaide Hospital Society continues to have a special relationship with the Faculty of Health Sciences in Trinity College Dublin in the recruitment of students for the degree programme. (5.39)

The Commission recommends that interview procedures are carefully formulated to obtain universal standards within each discipline whilst allowing interviewers determine the vocational commitment and suitability of applicants. (5.40)

The Commission recommends that the Board have the responsibility of overseeing the interview process in the selection of candidates for the degree programme. (5.41)

The Commission recommends that the Board keep the systems used in the selection of students for nursing under constant review to ensure the continuing use of best practice. The cost of administering the selection process should be met by the State. (5.41)

The Commission recommends that the student nursing grant and any student benefits for students on the proposed pre-registration nursing degree programme should be the same as those available to other third-level students and be means tested. (5.43)

The Commission recommends that the student is paid a salary during the twelve months continuous clinical placement at the level of eighty percent of the first year staff nurse's salary. This is the current level of payment for third year apprenticeship students. The twelve months continuous clinical placement for which a student is paid should be subsequently reckonable for pension purposes. Following graduation, the Commission recommends that a nurse, who has completed the twelve months continuous clinical placement, should start employment at the second increment point on the staff nurse salary scale. (5.44)

The Commission recommends that mature students should have a certain percentage of the third-level places in nursing assigned to them. The Commission recommends the percentage be determined by the third-level institutes in consultation with the Board. (5.45)

The Commission recommends a bursary/sponsorship system be put in place by the Department of Health and Children to promote applications to all disciplines by mature students. (5.46)

The Commission recommends that the Board and the Department of Health and Children examine mechanisms of promoting the profession as a career option among school leavers. (5.47)

The Commission recommends that the Board examine mechanisms of increasing the number of male candidates applying to enter the profession. (5.48)

The Commission recommends that health service employers consult with each nurse tutor currently involved in pre-registration nursing education in relation to her or his desired future career pathway. The purpose of the consultation is to establish whether the tutor wishes to move into third-level education or pursue other avenues in continuing education within the health service or other career options in management or clinical practice. The Commission recommends that health service providers support nurse tutors in upgrading their educational or other qualifications to facilitate their transition to their desired career pathway. (5.57)

The Commission recommends, in order to facilitate the transition of as many nurse tutors as possible to the third-level sector, that those nurse tutors who may not have been successful in competing for academic posts within third-level institutes or who do not meet the academic and other requirements for appointment as a lecturer within the academic career structure of a third-level institute be appointed as "nurse lecturers" on a personal basis in a similar manner to that developed in Northern Ireland. (5.58)

The Commission recommends that following the transition of pre-registration nursing education to a third-level degree programme, future nurse educators be appointed within the academic career structure of a third-level institute. (5.59)

The Commission recommends that in the transfer to a university/college-based degree programme there should be a number of joint appointments between third-level institutes and health service providers. (5.60)

The Commission recommends that the schools of nursing become centres of nursing education providing a range of educational and training services to nurses in the health services. (5.61)

The Commission recommends that clinical placement co-ordinators be retained to ensure the quality of clinical placements and the suitability of clinical areas to which students are assigned during clinical placements. The Commission recommends that there be a national evaluation of the role of the clinical placement co-ordinator and the continued development of the post. (5.65)

The Commission recommends that the posts of Practice Development Co-ordinator be given explicit further responsibility to develop clinical nursing research within a health service provider. (5.67)

The Commission recommends that practice development co-ordinators oversee the organisation of the pre-registration clinical placements. In order to fulfil the proposed combination of educational, management and research functions required in the Practice Development Co-ordinator posts the Commission recommends that future appointees to the post be educated to masters degree level. (5.67)

Professional Development

6.1   This chapter considers professional development issues in nursing and midwifery. The Commission is aware of the absolute importance of continuing education to the quality of services offered to patients and the development and growth of professional nursing and midwifery. Central to this is the development of a framework for continuing education and a clinical career pathway for nurses and midwives. The chapter is divided into four sections which deal with issues arising from the consultative process, continuing professional education, the development of a clinical career pathway for nurses and midwives and research in nursing and midwifery.

Issues Arising from the Consultative Process

6.2   Chapter four of the Commission on Nursing's interim report identified the important professional development issues facing nurses and midwives. The main issues have been outlined below.

6.3   Deficiencies in the ability of the profession to respond in an effective and proactive manner to the ever increasing pace of change and developments in the health services were highlighted in submissions made to the Commission. To address this issue, a comprehensive and coherent system of continuing professional education for nurses providing equity in access, availability of programmes and funding for courses was called for by nurses and midwives.

6.4   The Commission received submissions from approximately sixty groups and individual nurses who consider themselves to be "specialists" in particular areas of nursing and midwifery practice. Many of these nursing or midwifery specialities operate alongside medical specialities and seem to have developed in response to demands from medical professionals for more specialised nurses or midwives to support the medical field. A further group of areas which might also be regarded as nursing or midwifery specialities appears to have developed in response to the demands for changes in nursing and midwifery practice.

6.5   Many requests were made to the Commission for support in developing expanded/extended new roles for nurses and midwives. Heretofore, specialist and new expanded roles have largely developed in an informal, unstructured manner and have not been developed within a clinical career pathway.

6.6   It was submitted that the field of nursing and midwifery knowledge and its associated skills have become too vast and complex for any one nurse or midwife to master in full. The Commission was asked to recognise that specialisation, developed within the framework of a clinical career pathway, is a necessity.

6.7   The proliferation of post-registration courses of varying length, content and academic award and the need for career guidance for nurses and midwives when selecting post-registration programmes was impressed on the Commission.

6.8   The interim report of the Commission identified the need for nursing and midwifery practice to be underpinned by research. There was a call for structures to be put in place which would encourage, support and develop nursing and midwifery research.

The Professional Development of Nurses and Midwives

6.9   This section sets out the proposed framework in relation to post-registration nursing and midwifery education, which deals with the establishment of a National Council for Professional Development in Nursing and Midwifery and a Nursing and Midwifery Planning and Development Unit for each health board area. The section also makes recommendations in relation to study leave.

6.10   The Commission, in considering a framework for post-registration/continuing nursing and midwifery education, gave particular consideration to the document produced by the Board, entitled *Continuing Professional Education for Nurses in Ireland: A Framework*, published in 1997 as well as the proposals contained in the submissions made to the Commission. Consideration was also given to the *National Review of Specialist Nurse Education* published by the Australian Government Publishing Service in 1997.

6.11   The Commission has adopted the following definition of continuing education which was embraced by the Board:

"Continuing education is a life long professional development process which takes place after the completion of the pre-registration nurse education programme. It consists of planned learning experiences which are designed to augment the knowledge, skills and attitudes of registered nurses for the enhancement of nursing practice, patient/client care, education, administration and research" (An Bord Altranais, 1994).

The Commission sees the need to develop and strengthen the availability of professional development for all nurses and midwives. The Commission suggests that it might be helpful to consider professional development under the following three broad headings:

- in-service training - which might, for example, consist of education on occupational health issues and work orientation programmes;

- continuing education - which might consist of education on developments in nursing and the treatment of patient groups; and

- specialist training - which would consist of dedicated educational programmes and experience, supporting a nurse seeking to practice at an advanced level.

The Commission recommends that the Minister for Health and Children (the Minister) make provision for the three main areas of professional development to be fostered and further developed.

6.12   The Commission is aware of the urgent need to give guidance and direction in relation to the development of specialist nursing and midwifery posts and post-registration educational programmes offered to nurses and midwives. The enormity of the task is acknowledged by the Commission and having considered the matter at some length, the view is that a special body (separate to the Board) should be formed to address this matter in a focused and expedient manner. To this end, **the Commission recommends the Minister establish an independent statutory agency with responsibility for post-registration professional development of nursing and midwifery. The Commission recommends the independent statutory agency be called the National Council for the Professional Development of Nursing and Midwifery (the National Council).**

6.13   The Commission envisages that the Board would concentrate on entry to nursing and midwifery, on-going monitoring of the registration/diploma course, the development of pre-registration nursing degree programmes, giving professional leadership and providing an ethical framework for the development of professional practice. The Board would fulfil the important role of setting the professional standards and defining scope of practice. The National Council would concentrate on giving guidance to the profession in relation to the development of specialist nursing and midwifery posts, in addition to accrediting post-registration courses which prepare nurses and midwives for specialist practice.

National Council for Professional Development in Nursing and Midwifery

6.14   As stated previously, the Commission recommends that the Minister establish the National Council as a statutory body, with its own officers. *The Commission recommends the National Council be given the following functions:*

To:

- *monitor the on-going development of nursing and midwifery specialities, taking into account, changes in practice and service need;*

- *establish guidelines for the creation of specialist nursing and midwifery posts by health service providers;*

- *determine the appropriate level of qualification and experience for entry into specialist nursing and midwifery practice (interim and long-term requirements);*

- *accredit specialist nursing and midwifery courses (including those provided independently by universities and colleges) for the purpose of appointment as a clinical nurse or midwife specialist or advanced nurse or midwife practitioner, taking account of: standards of professional practice and conduct set by the Board; geographic spread and access by nurses and midwives; and, in particular, service need;*

- *support additional developments in continuing nurse education by health boards and voluntary organisations;*

- *assist health service providers by setting guidelines for the selection of nurses and midwives who might apply for financial support in seeking opportunities to pursue further education;*

- *accredit post-registration courses (other than those courses leading to registration as a midwife, public health nurse, sick children's nurse or nurse tutor) for the purpose of recording on the register maintained by the Board;*

- *liaise with bodies in other jurisdictions in relation to the professional development of nursing and midwifery; and*

- *publish an annual report on its activities, including the disbursement of monies by the Council.*

6.15   It is envisaged that the National Council will approve courses to ensure accessibility, a geographic spread in the provision of specialist courses, as well as maximise the use of educational resources. The National Council would also develop a comprehensive database in relation to the provision of specialist post-registration nursing and midwifery education. It would also determine the appropriate level of qualification and experience for entry into speciality practice.

6.16   In its deliberations on a post-registration course, the National Council should engage in on-going consultations with the Board on the proposed practice outcomes of the course in relation to professional standards and scope of practice guidelines. In addition, the two members of the Board nominated as members of the National Council (see paragraph 6.19) should provide advice and guidance on issues relating to professional standards. Finally, the National Council should notify the Board in writing of its intention to accredit a post-registration course, outlining the practice outcomes of the course. The National Council will accredit the course unless, within thirty days of the issuing of the notification from the Council, the Board informs the National Council in writing that in its view the practice outcomes of the course are not within the parameters of professional standards and scope of practice guidelines.

6.17 **The Commission recommends that the National Council be funded through the Department of Health and Children** to assist health service providers financially in the development of specialist training and continuing nurse education programmes. The National Council would support additional developments in continuing nurse education by health boards and voluntary organisations. The National Council could also retain some discretionary funding to contribute to the organisation of seminars on professional issues by other organisations.

6.18 **The Commission recommends that:**

- **the National Council have a board of twenty members appointed by the Minister for a five year period;**

- **members be limited to serving two consecutive terms on the National Council; of the first National Council appointed by the Minister, half of the membership be limited to serving one term of office;**

- **on the first National Council appointed by the Minister, members limited to serving one term be selected by lottery on appointment;**

- **the Chair be appointed by the Minister and that subsequent Chairs be elected by the members of the board; and**

- **the Chair have a five year term of office.**

6.19 **The Commission recommends that the Minister provide for the following membership of the council:**

- **seven registered nurses, one from each of the following areas: general nursing, mental handicap nursing, psychiatric nursing, public health nursing, sick children's nursing, care of the elderly and a nurse tutor. The nurses appointed by the Minister from the various disciplines must be nurses of high professional standing with experience of advanced practice;**

- **a registered midwife of high professional standing with experience of advanced practice;**

- **two members of An Bord Altranais nominated by the Board;**

- **one member following consultation with the Office for Health Management;**

- **one senior nurse manager following consultation with the appropriate professional bodies;**

- **two members following consultation with the Health Service Employers Agency;**

- **two officers of the Department of Health and Children, one of whom shall be the Chief Nursing Officer at the Department;**

- **one medical practitioner following consultation with the Royal College of Surgeons, the Royal College of Physicians, the Irish College of General Practitioners and the Royal College of Psychiatrists in Ireland; and**

- **three nurses or midwives following consultation with third-level institutes, one of whom shall be the Head of a Department of Nursing in a NUI University, one shall be the Head of a Department of Nursing in a non-NUI University and one shall be the Head of a Department of Nursing in an Institute of Technology or a Regional Technical College.**

Nursing and Midwifery Planning and Development Units

6.20   In considering the management of the health services, the **Commission recommends the establishment of a Nursing and Midwifery Planning and Development Unit at health board level** (see chapter seven). It is envisaged that part of the role of the unit would include overseeing the provision of continuing nursing and midwifery education for the health board area.

These units would have the following general functions:

- strategic planning and quality assurance of nursing and midwifery services in a health board area;

- co-ordinating the delivery of nursing and midwifery services and improving co-operation between health board and voluntary bodies in the delivery of nursing and midwifery services;

- liaising with centres of nursing education in the provision of continuing education for nurses within the health board area;

- working in partnership with the Chief Nursing Officer in the Department of Health and Children in planning/policy development of nursing and midwifery issues; and

- assisting in improving internal communications with nurses and midwives in a health board area.

6.21   In relation to continuing education, the **Commission recommends that the Nursing and Midwifery Planning and Development Units would have responsibility for overseeing the detailed provision of continuing nursing and midwifery education within a health board area.** Such provision could range from running day seminars within individual institutions, to supporting nurses and midwives to undertake specialist education on courses accredited by the National Council. These units would also have a role in fostering nursing and midwifery research at health board level.

6.22   The Nursing and Midwifery Policy and Development Units would submit development plans to the National Council when applying for additional development funding to support continuing nursing and midwifery education. These plans could be approved and funded by the National Council for up to three year periods. Fees, in respect of post-registration courses or bursaries to support students on post-registration courses, would be paid by the Nursing and Midwifery Planning and Development Units according to the guidelines laid down by the National Council.

Study Leave for Continuing Education

6.23   **The Commission recommends the Minister provide that the contract of employment of every nurse and midwife, in the public service, should entitle them to release, by an employer, for a minimum of two days paid study leave each year for continuing professional education.** With agreement from employers, such leave could be accumulated over three years. A nurse or midwife would be required by an employer to maintain a profile of professional development and show proof of attendance at seminars or conferences relevant to nursing or midwifery practice in utilising the two days paid study leave each year. **The Commission recommends that the proprietors of nursing homes assist their nursing staff in updating practice by providing for two days paid study leave for continuing education each year.** The Commission acknowledges that the implementation of this recommendation will have financial implications for health service providers.

Clinical Career Pathway

6.24   The consultative process identified the need for order and a coherent approach to the progression of specialisation and the development of a clinical career pathway for nursing and midwifery. This important function would form a large component of the work of the proposed National Council and the Nursing and Midwifery Planning and Development Unit in each health board area (referred to earlier in this chapter). The Commission is making recommendations for the development of a clinical career pathway from two perspectives; the long-term vision of the established clinical career path and the interim arrangements that will be required to reach this position.

6.25   The Commission has used the following information sources when considering the issue of a clinical career pathway: submissions made to the Commission; a review of the Irish and international literature; advice from the Board and Irish Nurse Managers and Educators; site visits in Australia to review the work of clinical nurse specialists (CNSs) and clinical nurse consultants (CNCs); advice of Australian nurse managers, nurse educators, The New South Wales Nurses Regulatory Body, The Australian College of Nurses and The Council of Deans of Nursing in Australia; the UKCC guidelines in relation to Post-registration Education and Practice (PREP) and advice from the Chair of the UKCC group reviewing the development of specialist and advanced practice in nursing in the UK.

6.26   The Commission is of the view that promotional opportunities should be open to nurses and midwives who wish to remain in clinical practice rather than following a management or education path. Currently, there is no career pathway for nurses wishing to advance their practice in clinical nursing and midwifery. *The Commission recommends the establishment of a multi-stage pathway for clinical nursing and midwifery and in particular, recommends that the Minister provide for a three step clinical career path in nursing and midwifery. The Commission recommends the following clinical career pathway:*

- *registered nurse/midwife;*

- *clinical nurse or midwife specialist (CNS) - equivalent to ward sister level; and*

- *advanced nurse or midwife practitioner (ANP) - equivalent to middle nursing and midwifery management level.*

The terms and conditions of employment should be determined through the normal channels.

6.27   It is not intended that there would be automatic progression through each step of the clinical career ladder. Seniority or years of clinical experience alone would not entitle a nurse or midwife to promotion. *The Commission recommends that for progression along the clinical career ladder, nurses and midwives must meet the practice and education guidelines set by the National Council.* Although not formally recognised today, there are several nurses and midwives operating in roles that could be described as those of clinical nurse or midwife specialists. The development of the position of advanced nurse or midwife practitioner is also currently emerging in Ireland; however, very few posts have yet been established. It is anticipated that in the future it would be a requirement for nurses or midwives appointed to the post of advanced nurse or midwife practitioner to have first held the post of a clinical specialist. Advanced nurse or midwife practitioner posts should be developed to meet future service needs.

6.28   There is a difference between a nurse or midwife working within a speciality area and the work of a nurse or midwife specialist. This view has been emphasised by the UKCC, the International Council for Nurses (ICN) and the Board. It does not necessarily follow that nurses or midwives, with specialist post-registration qualifications working in specialist areas such as accident and emergency departments or neonatal intensive care, are clinical nurse or midwife specialists. The role envisaged for the clinical nurse or midwife specialists (CNSs) is very specific and differs largely from that of the registered nurse or midwife involved in the day-to-day delivery of services. A nurse or midwife working in a speciality area operating at the primary practice level is not a clinical nurse or midwife specialist.

6.29 *The Commission recommends that to use either the title of "clinical nurse or midwife specialist" or "advanced nurse or midwife practitioner", a nurse or midwife must be appointed to a particular post. The recognition of CNS and ANP status must be matched with specified posts within the health services.*

6.30 *The Commission recommends that the Minister provide for a grade of clinical nurse or midwife specialist equivalent to ward sister level. The Commission recommends that the Minister also provide for a grade of advanced nurse or midwife practitioner equivalent to middle nursing and midwifery management level. The terms and conditions of employment should be determined through the normal channels.*

6.31 Because of the variety of health care delivery models, (both in hospitals and in the community), it is not possible to be prescriptive in relation to the appropriate reporting relationships for CNSs and ANPs. The precise arrangements will vary from one organisation to another. *The Commission recommends that the reporting relationships for each CNS and ANP be identified when the post is being established.* The job description for each post should clearly state the particular reporting mechanism. It is anticipated, that where appropriate in large acute hospitals, CNSs might report to the unit nursing officer/services manager or assistant director of nursing for the particular area. However it is essential that close collaborative relationships are maintained between CNSs/ANPs and first line nurse managers (clinical nurse managers) at unit/ward level or in the community.

Guidelines for Clinical Nurse Specialist and Advanced Nurse Practitioner Roles

6.32 *The Commission recommends that the National Council takes a lead role in defining and differentiating between the role of the CNS and ANP.* The Commission is aware of international difficulties encountered in this matter. To start the work, the Commission recommends the following guidelines for nurses wishing to take future posts as CNSs or ANPs. The guidelines outlined have been informed by international developments in the area, most notably in Australia, in the *National Review of Specialist Nurse Education* (1997) and the UKCC developments since the launch of the framework document *Post-Registration Education and Practice* (PREP) in 1994.

Clinical Nurse or Midwife Specialist

6.33 The literature reviews conducted on behalf of the Commission have been used to assist the Commission in formulating initial guidelines for the development of clinical nurse or midwife specialist (CNS) posts in Ireland; these are set out below:

- the CNS should be prepared beyond the level of a generalist;

- the CNS should have extensive experience and advanced expertise in the relevant specialist area of nursing or midwifery;

- the CNS should have undertaken a formally recognised relevant specialist post-registration course of study, at the minimum level of university/college diploma. This course should provide theoretical instruction and substantial clinical experience to ensure competency in the speciality practice (in the interim, certificate level or some other form of qualification or experience might be acceptable, if approved by the National Council);

- the CNS will work with medical colleagues and/or interdisciplinary team members within a specified area;

- the CNS may make variations in prescribed clinical options, within agreed protocols; and

- speciality practice of the clinical nurse or midwife specialist includes clinical practice, teaching, research implementation and advisory roles (adapted from ICN, 1992).

Advanced Nurse or Midwife Practitioner

6.34 The Commission is aware of the various and differing interpretations for the "practitioner". For this reason the Commission recommends the use of the title advanced nurse or midwife practitioner in the clinical career ladder. An outline of the role envisaged for the ANP is given below. The ANP:

- exercises higher levels of judgement, discretion and decision making in the clinical area above that expected of the clinical nurse or midwife specialist;

- has extensive experience in the relevant area of nursing or midwifery;

- has undertaken advanced education in the relevant specialist area at masters degree level involving theoretical content and substantial clinical experience;

- receives clients with undifferentiated and undiagnosed problems and initiates treatments according to agreed protocols and within agreed parameters;

- practises an advanced expanded nursing or midwifery role, makes professionally autonomous decisions taking sole responsibility, within agreed protocols;

- works independently, but closely, with other professionals and respects professional boundaries; and

- monitors and improves standards of care and develops practice by active involvement in advanced clinical practice, carrying out audits, being involved in teaching patients and colleagues and conducting research.

6.35 From the guidelines outlined it is apparent that the distinguishing features between the CNS and the ANP are found in the level of educational preparation, independence in practice, autonomy in clinical treatments, level of research involvement and role in the education of future CNSs and ANPs.

Organisation of the Clinical Career Pathway

6.36 It is vitally important that the future clinical pathway for nursing is broad based. The clinical career pathway should include specialisation but must also equally apply to all disciplines and areas of nursing. Advanced practice nursing is as important in care of the elderly as it is in critical care nursing. This wider approach should minimise the concern that clinical career pathways might not develop in all nursing areas, a concern that was expressed by some nurses during the consultative process. *Where the work envisaged for the CNS does not support a full-time post, the Commission recommends that the nurse or midwife be facilitated to work time as a CNS and time as a registered nurse or midwife, as appropriate.*

6.37   The rapid development of new specialist and sub-specialist nursing roles within each discipline of nursing was identified in the submissions made to the Commission. There is a danger that the proliferation of such roles could lead to a fragmentation of the nursing service and difficulty in filling future specialist positions. There is also the risk of creating future career "cul de sacs" for nurses or midwives operating in very specialised areas. The Commission is aware of the importance of ensuring that the development of CNS and ANP posts is not confined to high technology areas or domains where advanced nursing or midwifery education is already well established.

6.38   These issues were examined by the national review body for specialist nurse education in Australia (1997). Following extensive consultation, the group recommended that the career structure for nursing be guided by seven broad band nomenclatures with related sub-specialties. These are: maternal and child health nursing; high dependency nursing; mental health nursing; rehabilitation and habilitation nursing (quality of life issues); medical/surgical nursing; community health nursing and functional nursing (management). The report envisaged that the broad band areas be used to give coherence to the development of specialist nursing posts and the direction of future post-registration educational programmes.

6.39   The Commission is suggesting that the Australian model be used as a guide and modified for the Irish nursing environment. *The Commission recommends the Minister provide that the clinical career path be organised around seven broad bands of nursing and midwifery. The seven suggested broad band nomenclatures which might be used to group the relevant sub-specialist areas are set out below. The examples of sub-specialist areas given for each broad band area are only for illustrative purposes. The National Council will determine the range of sub-specialist areas within each broad band nomenclature.*

- *high dependency nursing, (this broad band might include areas such as coronary care, intensive therapy (psychiatry) and neonatal intensive care nursing);*

- *rehabilitation and habilitation nursing, (this broad band might include areas such as care of the elderly, spinal injuries and palliative care nursing);*

- *medical/surgical nursing, (this broad band might include areas such as oncology, infection control, stoma care, neurosciences and anaesthesia nursing);*

- *maternal and child health nursing, (this broad band might include areas such as parent craft, ultrasonography, paediatric cardiology and paediatric oncology nursing);*

- *community health nursing, (this broad band might include areas such as health education and health promotion, family development and community psychiatry);*

- *mental health nursing, (this broad band might include areas such as addiction counselling and behaviour therapy); and*

- *disability nursing, (this broad band might include areas such as sensory stimulation and challenging behaviour).*

6.40   The suggested broad band areas are not intended to replace or add to the existing disciplines of nursing which currently lead to registration with the Board (these would continue unchanged). The intention is to give coherence and order to the multiple sub-specialist areas which have developed within each discipline. The broad band areas would fall under the recognised disciplines of nursing. At post-registration level high dependency nursing and the relevant sub-specialist areas could equally apply to general, sick children's, midwifery or psychiatric nursing. The strength of this framework is that it encompasses the needs of each of the disciplines of nursing (general, psychiatric, mental handicap, midwifery, sick children's and public health nursing).

6.41   The Commission is of the view that seven broad band nursing categories within the disciplines should offer greater flexibility to individual nurses and midwives when considering future career plans. The Commission envisages that the educational requirements would include common modules in the broad band area together with modules in the particular sub-specialty area. Nurses and midwives, working in very focused sub-specialist areas, will have the option of moving to related sub-specialist areas within their particular grouping. Having obtained the required educational qualification for one sub-specialist area within a particular broad band, the nurse or midwife could later be facilitated to move to another sub-specialist area by completing an additional module of education.

Education for Clinical Nurse Specialists and Advanced Nurse Practitioners

6.42   *The National Review of Specialist Nurse Education* (1997) reported that in Australia the proliferation of nursing specialities and the equally rapid development in educational provision has resulted in a lack of a unified scheme by which to determine requirements and qualifications for entry into particular areas of nursing speciality practice. This caused difficulties for employers when determining required qualifications for specialist staff, as well as for nurses and midwives in selecting their preferred career path. The Commission is aware of a similar proliferation of post-registration nursing courses in Ireland of varying length, content and academic award. Many of the Irish courses have an imbalance between theory and clinical practice. During the consultative process nurses expressed concern in relation to the availability and geographic accessibility of further education courses. There was a view that the "substantial" clinically-based specialist courses are only available in Dublin.

6.43   At present most specialist post-registration education courses, are provided by health service providers and small numbers are provided by university departments of nursing in partnership with health service providers. These courses are generally awarded Category Two approval by the Board. During most post-registration courses, the cohort of nurses forms part of the workforce in the specialist area and are released for the theoretical component of the programme. Successful candidates of hospital programmes are awarded a hospital certificate and those from university programmes are awarded a higher diploma in the specialist area of nursing. The hospital programmes are generally organised and co-ordinated by a nurse with clinical expertise in the area of practice, usually called a course co-ordinator or course facilitator. A nurse tutor is assigned overall responsibility for the programme.

6.44   The Commission suggests that the seven broad bands be used to guide the future post-graduate nursing educational developments in Ireland. Education providers for nursing and midwifery should be encouraged to ensure that advanced programmes are available in the broad band areas with modules to cater for the sub-specialist areas. Each education programme should comprise theoretical instruction and a significant amount of clinical practice.

6.45   In developing courses, third-level institutes must maintain close contact with health service providers and respond to their identified need to prepare nurses for particular specialist nursing roles. A coherent framework is required for the development of such education programmes, which must meet academic standards.

6.46   ***The Commission recommends that the development of post-registration programmes will take place following collaboration between:***

● ***the National Council for Professional Development in Nursing and Midwifery;***

● ***universities/third-level colleges; and***

- *health service providers and the centres of nursing education.*

6.47   It is envisaged that third-level institutes, in consultation with health service providers, would prepare curricula for university/college diplomas and masters degree programmes, which would prepare nurses for positions as CNSs or ANPs. The professional standards required by the Board and the guidelines of the National Council must be given careful attention when designing curricula for specialist programmes (see paragraph 6.16 of this chapter).

6.48   **The Commission recommends that education providers submit their curricula to the National Council for accreditation.** The accreditation process will ensure that the requirements of the National Council for professional recognition as a CNS or ANP are met. The National Council will co-ordinate the equal distribution of courses throughout the country, taking into account the local service needs. Nurses who have completed specialist education programmes, accredited by the National Council, will be eligible to apply for CNS and ANP posts.

6.49   Support for fees in respect of post-registration courses or bursaries to support students on post-registration courses would be funded through the Nursing and Midwifery Planning and Development Units. The National Council has a role in providing guidelines for the selection of nurses and midwives who might apply for financial support in seeking opportunities to pursue further education.

6.50   **The Commission recommends that programmes intending to prepare nurses and midwives for the role of CNS or ANP should have a large component of clinical practice (competency being assessed during the programme) and the programme should be accredited by the National Council.**

6.51   The Commission, in considering the future direction of post-registration nursing education, was conscious of the need to develop simultaneously a coherent framework for the nurse educators currently involved in the delivery of post-registration programmes; these include nurse tutors, course co-ordinators and course facilitators. **The Commission recommends the creation of joint clinical/academic appointments to establish strong links between theory and specialist clinical practice.**

6.52   **The Commission recommends that when negotiating the move of post-registration programmes to third-level institutes, health service employers undertake a detailed consultation with the nurse educators currently involved in post-registration education programmes. Each nurse educator should be consulted in relation to her or his desired future career pathway, whether she or he wishes to move into the third-level sector, pursue other avenues in professional development within the health service or other career options in management or clinical practice. The Commission recommends that health service providers support post-registration nurse educators in upgrading their education or other qualifications to facilitate their transition to their desired career pathway.**

6.53   As indicated in the guidelines given earlier in the document, **the Commission recommends that clinical nurse or midwife specialists undertake a relevant specialist post-registration university/college diploma and have extensive experience in the particular field of nursing or midwifery.** The Commission is conscious that there may be an initial practical difficulty for some nurses, as the specialist university/college diploma courses may not yet be available for their area of practice. In the interim, certificate level or some other form of qualification or experience may be acceptable. However, this is a matter for the National Council to consider in greater detail. In the longer-term it is anticipated that graduate nurses, wishing to pursue a career as a CNS, will obtain post-graduate diploma level qualifications. **The Commission recommends that advanced nurse or midwife practitioners, who will be expected to conduct research into clinical nursing or midwifery issues, be prepared to masters degree level.**

6.54   The Commission does not consider it appropriate for nurses who have not attained the prescribed educational level to be automatically appointed to CNS or ANP posts. This recommendation is based on the advice and experiences of Australian nurse managers when introducing a clinical career structure for nursing in Australia in the late 1980's. Some of the nurses appointed to posts at that time did not have advanced educational preparation, nor did they achieve it once confirmed in post. While currently holding clinical nurse specialist posts, it appears that some nurses are not operating at the advanced level expected of clinical nurse specialists.

6.55   It is important that Irish nurses and midwives, who have pioneered and led the development of nursing and midwifery without the benefit of advanced education (as it was not available at the time), are appreciated. *The Commission recommends that nurses and midwives with substantial specialist experience should be given accreditation for prior education and experience when seeking entry to specialist educational programmes.* They should be encouraged, supported and assisted (including financial assistance and study leave with replacement) by the health service to obtain the relevant educational qualification.

Establishing Clinical Nurse or Midwife Specialist and Advanced Nurse or Midwife Practitioner Posts

6.56   The consultative process clearly highlighted the urgent need to establish officially a clinical career path for nurses and midwives in Ireland. The first step in this process is to approve and set up, on a national basis, posts of clinical nurse or midwife specialists. A time scale for the establishment of the initial cohort of CNS and ANP positions must be agreed. This will involve reviewing existing posts (which heretofore have not been formally recognised as posts of CNS) and establishing new CNS posts in response to service needs. It is envisaged that a detailed analysis of both the local and national service needs will be required before the optimal numbers of CNS and ANP posts can be determined. The establishment of CNS and ANP posts should be based on the needs of the particular organisation and the services provided for patients. It is thought that the final number and areas of work would be determined following consultation between:

- the Director of Nursing/Chief Nursing Officer/Superintendent Public Health Nurse;

- the Chief Executive Officer (CEO) for the organisation;

- the Nurse Planning and Development Unit for the health board area and health board CEO;

- the National Council for Professional Development in Nursing and Midwifery; and

- the Department of Health and Children.

6.57   Senior nurses and midwives with extensive clinical experience, currently in practice, must be valued and encouraged to seek posts as CNSs or ANPs. To achieve this, they should be strongly encouraged and assisted to obtain the educational qualifications set out in the guidelines for CNS or ANP positions. In the interim, specialist clinical experience accompanied by certificate level qualifications may be acceptable when appointing CNSs. However, the interim measure should only apply to specialist certificate programmes approved by the National Council.

6.58   The Commission is aware that there are currently a number of nurses working in roles similar to those envisaged for the CNS or ANP, who have not had the opportunity to pursue specialist post-registration programmes (either certificate or diploma) because appropriate programmes are not available in Ireland. Nurses working in such positions will need particular consideration when the clinical career ladder is being developed. The interim arrangements should apply to nurses currently in specialist positions when the first cohort of CNS posts are being created. Thereafter the practice and education guidelines set out in paragraphs 6.33 and 6.34 of this chapter should apply. To be eligible to apply for CNS or ANP posts the nurse or midwife must have completed the relevant education programme which is accredited by the National Council.

6.59   *The Commission recommends the following process for creating CNS/ANP posts:*

- *the National Council would initially agree the guidelines - an interim set and long-term guidelines, for the recognition and establishment of the posts of clinical nurse or midwife specialist and advanced nurse or midwife practitioner;*

- *the Director of Nursing/Chief Nursing Officer/Superintendent Public Health Nurse, in consultation with nurse managers (first line and middle), would identify the need for developing a number of CNS and possibly ANP posts for specified areas within their own organisation;*

- *a detailed job description would be devised outlining the requirements (experience and education) specified by the National Council and the appropriate reporting relationship for the post holder;*

- *a plan for the development of such posts would be prepared (based on service needs and the criteria set down by the National Council and guidance from the Nursing and Midwifery Planning and Development Unit) for the health board area;*

- *the senior nurses and midwives for each organisation would submit their plans to the Nursing and Midwifery Planning and Development Unit;*

- *the plans and job specifications submitted would be reviewed by the Nursing and Midwifery Planning and Development Unit in consultation with senior nursing and general management. This would ensure that a cohesive plan for the regional development of posts was put forward;*

- *the agreed plans would be submitted for approval to the Chief Executive of the hospital or health board, as appropriate; and*

- *the hospital or health board would submit the plan to the Department of Health and Children for approval.*

6.60   *The Commission recommends the following arrangements for appointing CNSs and ANPs:*

- *following approval for the creation of CNS and ANP posts, the responsibility for appointing suitably qualified nurses would rest with each health service provider;*

- *in the initial filling of posts, where the recognition and establishment of a post or posts have been identified, those nurses and midwives practising at a specialist level, who satisfy the criteria established by the Council (credit being given for prior education and experience) and are currently carrying out the duties of the approved post, should be appointed as clinical nurse or midwife specialists;*

- *where this situation does not arise, the posts should be advertised as soon as the approval of the Department is obtained and interviews should be conducted without delay; and*

- *pending the provision of the requisite graduate courses, all nurses or midwives who are appointed in the initial filling of vacant posts must agree, as a condition of their appointment, to obtain the proposed educational qualifications within an agreed time frame. This provision does not apply to nurses or midwives who are merely confirmed in specialist posts. Credit should be given for prior education and experience.*

6.61   ***The Commission recommends that all concerned afford top priority to the creation of CNS and ANP posts.*** It is envisaged that the Department of Health and Children and the Nursing and Midwifery Planning and Development Unit in each health board area will take a proactive role in this matter.

6.62   The Nursing and Midwifery Planning and Development Unit would have the role of monitoring the development of CNS/ANP posts. This would include investigating failure to develop posts within a health board, in all areas of nursing and midwifery (where a service need is apparent) and making representation accordingly.

Senior Staff Nurses and Midwives

6.63   The clinical career pathway, recommended by the Commission, will in time create a substantial range of increased career opportunities for nurses and midwives. However, the Commission is also conscious that many excellent nurses and midwives may not wish to specialise and seek promotion within the clinical, educational or management framework. Staff nurses and midwives will remain primarily responsible for the delivery of high quality care to patients and clients of the health service.

6.64   It was suggested that there needed to be increased recognition for those senior staff nurses and midwives who have provided many years of high quality public service within the health care sector. Using the Benner Model of skill progression, many senior nurses and midwives, on the basis of their extensive experience, are regarded by their colleagues as proficient/expert in their area of practice. There was a view expressed during the consultative process that senior staff nurses and midwives should have a further long service increment at some later stage in their career which would recognise their many years of contribution to the delivery of health services, without impacting on any differential. Similarly, there was a view that the annual leave entitlement of staff nurses and midwives should be on an incremental basis. It was argued that almost every other profession and occupation in the health services had a system of incremental annual leave according to the number of years service. It was stated that nursing and midwifery were physically arduous and emotionally stressful. The physical and stressful nature of nursing and midwifery, it was suggested, required a system of incremental annual leave to avoid "burn-out" amongst older nurses and midwives. ***The Commission recommends that the question of additional recognition of long service for staff nurses be examined through the established structures.***

Allowances

6.65   An issue raised during the consultative process by nurses and midwives in workshops, and in particular by the Nursing Alliance in a written submission, was the question of the dual qualified scale and the location-based and qualification allowances. The dual qualified scale applies to nurses who hold two of the following registerable qualifications; general, psychiatric or mental handicap nursing. It does not apply to an additional registerable qualification in midwifery or sick children's nursing. The dual qualified scale is referred to in the Blue Book in the following terms:

"retention on a red-circled basis and personal to those nurses who are paid on the dual qualified scale on 1st October 1996, and for those in appropriate post-graduate training on that date only. The issue of dual qualified nurse is to be returned to as part of phase 2 under the 'services requirements' element."

6.66   There are also location-based or qualification allowances which are paid to all nurses or midwives working in certain areas such as care of the elderly and intensive care. The Blue Book refers to the finding by the Adjudication Board that: *"the location-based and qualification allowances should continue* *to be paid to all nurses qualifying for same until revised arrangements are agreed between the parties on this issue".* A case was also made during the consultative process for recognition of extra qualifications which are attained by nurses and midwives. It was argued that the additional qualifications have a beneficial impact on patient care and there should be recognition given to the nurse or midwife which reflects this benefit to service. Having considered the matter, the Commission was of the view that the forum in which these claims should be addressed is properly the Labour Court.

The Commission recommends that outstanding claims for allowances should be referred to the Labour Court for argument and determination as a matter of urgency.

Segmentation of the Grade

6.67   One of the terms of reference for the Commission was "segmentation of the grade". The Commission understands this to mean the division of a grade into different levels as has happened in the United Kingdom in the staff nurse grade. As detailed earlier in the chapter, the Commission has recommended the creation of two new posts in clinical nursing (CNS and ANP posts). These are new promotional opportunities for clinical nurses and midwives and should not be confused with segmentation of the grade. The Commission does not recommend segmentation of the grade of staff nurse.

Nursing and Midwifery Research

6.68   The literature reviews conducted on behalf of the Commission identified a dearth of published Irish nursing and midwifery research. The Commission attaches a particular importance to the development of nursing and midwifery research at every level; within each individual organisation (hospital or community), at health board level and within the Department of Health and Children.

6.69   In *Continuing Professional Education: A Framework* (An Bord Altranais, 1997) it was suggested that nursing and midwifery research might form one of the four professional pathways for nursing and midwifery. However, the Commission is of the view that for nursing and midwifery practice to be evidence-based, research should form an integral part of all aspects of nursing and midwifery. For this reason, the **Commission recommends that nurses and midwives wishing to develop careers in research be encouraged and supported to do so through the clinical, education or management pathway.**

6.70   There is a need for nursing research to be promoted in clinical practice. Within organisations, the posts of practice development co-ordinators (described in Chapter Five) and advanced nurse practitioners (as outlined in 6.34 of this chapter) will make an important contribution, by instigating and leading research projects which examine clinical nursing and midwifery issues. The university sector, in collaboration with the health services, has an important role to play in the development of nursing and midwifery research. **The Commission recommends the creation of joint clinical/academic appointments to establish stronger research links between theory and practice and enhance the credibility of nursing and midwifery research.**

6.71   The investigation of patient care issues involves formal research specifically related to nursing and midwifery practice. The role requires a practice climate of clinical inquiry, critical thinking, formal research investigation and the ability to interpret, evaluate and communicate the findings. The title "Nurse Researcher" should be reserved for nurses involved in researching nursing issues and not given to those involved in data collection for medical or other research.

6.72   *The Commission recommends that the Minister provide for nursing and midwifery research to be funded through the Health Research Board (HRB)* thus ensuring that nursing and midwifery research is seen in the context of the overall research activity of the health services and maintains a high level of quality. *The Commission recommends that the Minister make funding available to the HRB specifically for nursing and midwifery research.*

6.73   *The Commission recommends that the Health Research Board establish a nursing and midwifery research advisory division which could assist and advise nurses and midwives on the presentation of projects for financial grants.*

6.74   *The Commission recommends that a comprehensive database of Irish nursing and midwifery research, funded by the State, be established.* Proposals for the operation of the database should be submitted to The Department of Health and Children.

6.75   *The Commission* attaches great importance to nursing and midwifery representation on the Health Research Board and *recommends that the Minister appoint a registered nurse or midwife, with experience in research, to the HRB*.

6.76   If nursing and midwifery research is to develop, it is important that efforts are made to ensure the education and development of nurse researchers, who will carry out research in nursing and midwifery which will stand up to rigorous academic analysis. A welcome development was made by the Board in September 1997 when they launched doctoral scholarships in nursing/midwifery, setting aside significant funding to support the scholarships. It is also noted from the annual report of the HRB for 1996, that eight advanced post doctoral research fellowships were awarded. The HRB, in conjunction with the Board, could in the future operate a scheme to support the development of nurses to Ph.D level, thus supporting the development of a cohort of high calibre nurse researchers.

6.77   To ensure a coherence in the development of nursing and midwifery research, it is the view of the Commission that the Nursing and Midwifery Policy Unit in the Department of Health and Children, in consultation with appropriate bodies, should draw up a national strategy for nursing and midwifery research. A strong recommendation on nursing research was made by the Committee of Ministers of Member States of the European Union in Document No R96(1). The Committee of Ministers, under Article 15.b of the Statute of the Council of Europe recommended that member states establish a strategy for the development of nursing research.

Summary

6.78   Central to the continued development of professional nursing is the enhancement of continuing professional education, the establishment of a clinical career pathway and the development of a strong body of skilled nurse researchers equipped to investigate clinical nursing issues. The provision of a minimum of two days paid study leave for every nurse and midwife is an important first step in ensuring equity and access to ongoing education. The establishment of the National Council for Professional Development in Nursing and Midwifery and the Nursing and Midwifery Planning and Development Unit in each health board are key to the development of a post-registration education framework and the establishment of the clinical career pathway. *The Commission recommends that as the profession develops and the career pathway is firmly established the arrangements set out in this chapter be reviewed.*

Summary of Recommendations in Chapter Six

The Commission recommends that the Minister for Health and Children (the Minister) make provision for the three main areas of professional development (in-service training, continuing education and specialist training) to be fostered and further developed. (6.11)

The Commission recommends the Minister establish an independent statutory agency with responsibility for post-registration professional development of nursing and midwifery. The Commission recommends the independent statutory agency be called the National Council for the Professional Development of Nursing and Midwifery (the National Council). (6.12)

The Commission recommends the National Council be given the following functions:

To:

- monitor the on-going development of nursing and midwifery specialities, taking into account changes in practice and service need;

- establish guidelines for the creation of specialist nursing and midwifery posts by health service providers;

- determine the appropriate level of qualification and experience for entry into specialist nursing and midwifery practice (interim and long-term requirements);

- accredit specialist nursing and midwifery courses (including those provided independently by universities and colleges) for the purpose of appointment as a clinical nurse or midwife specialist or advanced nurse or midwife practitioner, taking account of: standards of professional practice and conduct set by the Board; geographic spread and access by nurses and midwives; and, in particular, service need;

- support additional developments in continuing nurse education by health boards and voluntary organisations;

- assist health service providers by setting guidelines for the selection of nurses and midwives who might apply for financial support in seeking opportunities to pursue further education;

- accredit post-registration courses (other than those courses leading to registration as a midwife, public health nurse, sick children's nurse or nurse tutor) for the purpose of recording on the register maintained by the Board;

- liaise with bodies in other jurisdictions in relation to the professional development of nursing and midwifery; and

- publish an annual report on its activities, including the disbursement of monies by the Council. (6.14)

The Commission recommends that the National Council be funded through the Department of Health and Children. (6.17)

The Commission recommends that:

- the National Council have a board of twenty members appointed by the Minister for a five year period;

- members be limited to serving two consecutive terms on the National Council; of the first National Council appointed by the Minister, half of the membership be limited to serving one term of office;

- on the first National Council appointed by the Minister, members limited to serving one term be selected by lottery on appointment;

- the Chair be appointed by the Minister and that subsequent Chairs be elected by the members of the board; and

- the Chair have a five year term of office. (6.18)

The Commission recommends that the Minister provide for the following membership of the council:

- seven registered nurses, one from each of the following areas: general nursing, mental handicap nursing, psychiatric nursing, public health nursing, sick children's nursing, care of the elderly and a nurse tutor. The nurses appointed by the Minister from the various disciplines must be nurses of high professional standing with experience of advanced practice;

- a registered midwife of high professional standing with experience of advanced practice;

- two members of An Bord Altranais nominated by the Board;

- one member following consultation with the Office for Health Management;

- one senior nurse manager following consultation with the appropriate professional bodies;

- two members following consultation with the Health Service Employers Agency;

- two officers of the Department of Health and Children, one of whom shall be the Chief Nursing Officer at the Department;

- one medical practitioner following consultation with the Royal College of Surgeons, the Royal College of Physicians, the Irish College of General Practitioners and the Royal College of Psychiatrists in Ireland; and

- three nurses or midwives following consultation with third-level institutes, one of whom shall be the Head of a Department of Nursing in a NUI University, one shall be the Head of a Department of Nursing in a non-NUI University and one shall be the Head of a Department of Nursing in an Institute of Technology or a Regional Technical College. (6.19)

The Commission recommends the establishment of a Nursing and Midwifery Planning and Development Unit at health board level. (6.20)

The Commission recommends that the Nursing and Midwifery Planning and Development Units (recommended in chapter seven of the report) would have responsibility for overseeing the detailed provision of continuing nursing and midwifery education within a health board area. (6.21)

The Commission recommends the Minister provide that the contract of employment of every nurse and midwife, in the public service, should entitle them to release, by an employer, for a minimum of two days paid study leave each year for continuing professional education. (6.23)

The Commission recommends that the proprietors of nursing homes assist their nursing staff in updating practice by providing for two days paid study leave for continuing education each year. (6.23)

The Commission recommends the establishment of a multi-stage pathway for clinical nursing and midwifery and in particular, recommends that the Minister provide for a three step clinical career path in nursing and midwifery. The Commission recommends the following clinical career pathway:

- registered nurse/midwife;

- clinical nurse or midwife specialist (CNS) - equivalent to ward sister level; and

- advanced nurse or midwife practitioner (ANP) - equivalent to middle nursing and midwifery management level.

The terms and conditions of employment should be determined through the normal channels. (6.26)

The Commission recommends that for progression along the clinical career ladder, nurses and midwives must meet the practice and education guidelines set by the National Council. (6.27)

The Commission recommends that to use either the title of "clinical nurse or midwife specialist" or "advanced nurse or midwife practitioner", a nurse or midwife must be appointed to a particular post. The recognition of CNS and ANP status must be matched with specified posts within the health services. (6.29)

The Commission recommends that the Minister provide for a grade of clinical nurse or midwife specialist equivalent to ward sister level. The Commission recommends that the Minister also provide for a grade of advanced nurse or midwife practitioner equivalent to middle nursing and midwifery management level. The terms and conditions of employment should be determined through the normal channels. (6.30)

The Commission recommends that the reporting relationships for each CNS and ANP be identified when the post is being established. (6.31)

The Commission recommends that the National Council takes a lead role in defining and differentiating between the role of the CNS and ANP. (6.32)

Where the work envisaged for the CNS does not support a full-time post, the Commission recommends that the nurse or midwife be facilitated to work time as a CNS and time as a registered nurse or midwife, as appropriate. (6.36)

The Commission recommends the Minister provide that the clinical career path be organised around seven broad bands of nursing and midwifery. The seven suggested broad band nomenclatures which might be used to group the relevant sub-specialist areas are set out below. The examples of sub-specialist areas given for each broad band area are only for illustrative purposes. The National Council will determine the range of sub-specialist areas within each broad band nomenclature.

- high dependency nursing, (this broad band might include areas such as coronary care, intensive therapy (psychiatry) and neonatal intensive care nursing);

- rehabilitation and habilitation nursing, (this broad band might include areas such as care of the elderly, spinal injuries and palliative care nursing);

- medical/surgical nursing, (this broad band might include areas such as oncology, infection control, stoma care, neurosciences and anaesthesia nursing);

- maternal and child health nursing, (this broad band might include areas such as parent craft, ultrasonography, paediatric cardiology and paediatric oncology nursing);

- community health nursing, (this broad band might include areas such as health education and health promotion, family development and community psychiatry);

- mental health nursing, (this broad band might include areas such as addiction counselling and behaviour therapy); and

- disability nursing, (this broad band might include areas such as sensory stimulation and challenging behaviour). (6.39)

The Commission recommends that the development of post-registration programmes will take place following collaboration between:

- the National Council for Professional Development in Nursing and Midwifery;

- universities/third-level colleges; and

- health service providers and the centres of nursing education. (6.46)

The Commission recommends that education providers submit their curricula to the National Council for accreditation. (6.48)

The Commission recommends that programmes intending to prepare nurses and midwives for the role of CNS or ANP should have a large component of clinical practice (competency being assessed during the programme) and the programme should be accredited by the National Council. (6.50)

The Commission recommends the creation of joint clinical/academic appointments to establish strong links between theory and specialist clinical practice. (6.51)

The Commission recommends that when negotiating the move of post-registration programmes to third-level institutes, health service employers undertake a detailed consultation with the nurse educators currently involved in post-registration education programmes. Each nurse educator should be consulted in relation to her or his desired future career pathway whether she or he wishes to move into the third-level sector, pursue other avenues in professional development within the health service or other career options in management or clinical practice. The Commission recommends that health service providers support post-registration nurse educators in upgrading their education or other qualification to facilitate their transition to their desired career pathway. (6.52)

The Commission recommends that clinical nurse or midwife specialists undertake a relevant specialist post-registration university/college diploma and have extensive experience in the particular field of nursing or midwifery. (6.53)

The Commission recommends that advanced nurse or midwife practitioners, who will be expected to conduct research into clinical nursing or midwifery issues, be prepared to masters degree level. (6.53)

The Commission recommends that nurses and midwives with substantial specialist experience should be given accreditation for prior education and experience when seeking entry to specialist educational programmes. (6.55)

The Commission recommends the following process for creating CNS/ANP posts:

- the National Council would initially agree the guidelines - an interim set and long-term guidelines, for the recognition and establishment of the posts of clinical nurse or midwife specialist and advanced nurse or midwife practitioner;

- the Director of Nursing/Chief Nursing Officer/Superintendent Public Health Nurse, in consultation with nurse managers (first line and middle), would identify the need for developing a number of CNS and possibly ANP posts for specified areas within their own organisation;

- a detailed job description would be devised outlining the requirements (experience and education) specified by the National Council and the appropriate reporting relationship for the post holder;

- a plan for the development of such posts would be prepared (based on service needs and the criteria set down by the National Council and guidance from the Nursing and Midwifery Planning and Development Unit) for the health board area;

- the senior nurses and midwives for each organisation would submit their plans to the Nursing and Midwifery Planning and Development Unit;

- the plans and job specifications submitted would be reviewed by the Nursing and Midwifery Planning and Development Unit in consultation with senior nursing and midwifery and general management. This would ensure that a cohesive plan for the regional development of posts was put forward;

- the agreed plans would be submitted for approval to the Chief Executive of the hospital or health board, as appropriate; and

- the hospital or health board would submit the plan to the Department of Health and Children for approval. (6.59)

The Commission recommends the following arrangements for appointing CNSs and ANPs:

- following approval for the creation of CNS and ANP posts, the responsibility for appointing suitably qualified nurses would rest with each health service provider;

- in the initial filling of posts, where the recognition and establishment of a post or posts have been identified, those nurses and midwives practising at specialist level, who satisfy the criteria established by the Council (credit being given for prior education and experience) and are currently carrying out the duties of the approved post, should be appointed as clinical nurse or midwife specialists;

- where this situation does not arise, the posts should be advertised as soon as the approval of the Department is obtained and interviews should be conducted without delay; and

- pending the provision of the requisite graduate courses, all nurses or midwives who are appointed in the initial filling of vacant posts must agree, as a condition of their appointment, to obtain the proposed educational qualifications within an agreed time frame. This provision does not apply to nurses or midwives who are merely confirmed in specialist posts. Credit should be given for prior education and experience. (6.60)

The Commission recommends that all concerned afford top priority to the creation of CNS and ANP posts. (6.61)

The Commission recommends that the question of additional recognition of long service for staff nurses be examined through the established structures. (6.64)

The Commission recommends that outstanding claims for allowances should be referred to the Labour Court for argument and determination as a matter of urgency. (6.66)

The Commission recommends that nurses and midwives wishing to develop careers in research be encouraged and supported to do so through the clinical, education or management pathway. (6.69)

The Commission recommends the creation of joint clinical/academic appointments to establish stronger research links between theory and practice and enhance the credibility of nursing and midwifery research. (6.70)

The Commission recommends that the Minister provide for nursing and midwifery research to be funded through the Health Research Board (HRB). The Commission recommends that the Minister make funding available to the HRB specifically for nursing and midwifery research. (6.72)

The Commission recommends that the Health Research Board establish a nursing and midwifery research advisory division which could assist and advise nurses and midwives on the presentation of projects for financial grants. (6.73)

The Commission recommends that a comprehensive database of Irish nursing and midwifery research, funded by the State, be established. (6.74)

The Commission recommends that the Minister appoint a registered nurse or midwife with experience in research, to the HRB. (6.75)

The Commission recommends that as the profession develops and the career pathway is firmly established the arrangements set out in this chapter be reviewed. (6.78)

The Role of Nurses and Midwives in the Management of Services

7.1   This chapter outlines concerns identified during the consultative process in relation to the role of nurses and midwives in the management of the health services. These concerns related to a sense of exclusion from the strategic planning process, communication with nurses and midwives within organisations, the management of nursing and midwifery and the development of management potential within nursing and midwifery. The Commission recommends a framework for the greater inclusion of nursing and midwifery in the strategic planning process, the strengthening of nursing and midwifery management and the development of nurses and midwives for the management of nursing and midwifery within the wider health service. This chapter focuses on general issues in relation to the management of nursing and midwifery whilst making a number of recommendations specific to acute nursing and midwifery services. Chapter eight, Nursing in the Community, outlines the proposals of the Commission in relation to nursing management structures in the community, in particular, the development of the public health nursing management structure.

7.2   The role of nurses and midwives in the management of services must be seen in the context of increasing demands on the Irish health services in recent years. These demands have arisen from social and demographic changes in Irish society, the increasing consumer movement, the continuing rapid technological development in health care and the on-going need to account for the effective use of available resources. It is an environment where increasing demands for the provision and development of services must be placed within determined expenditure limits. *Shaping a Healthier Future*, published by the Department of Health in 1994, encapsulates the changes that have taken place in the Irish health services in recent years. This environment requires skillful management by all those with a management responsibility within the health services. As a consequence, the effective management of nursing and midwifery is particularly important because of the extent of the contact between patients/health service clients with nurses and midwives. The quality of care within the health service is primarily determined by the quality of the nursing and midwifery services. The effective management of the profession and the development of the nursing and midwifery management resource will have substantial benefits for the effective and efficient delivery of health care.

Issues Raised During the Consultative Process

7.3   A range of issues were identified during the consultative process in relation to the role of nurses and midwives in the management of services. These might be outlined as:

(i)   the need for greater internal communication within organisations;

(ii)   a perception that nurses/midwives and nursing/midwifery were not sufficiently involved in strategic planning or in policy development and strategy development;

(iii) the perception that there was a lack of partnership and consultation between general management and nursing/midwifery management and between nursing/midwifery management and nurses/midwives in the setting and attaining of corporate goals;

(iv)   a concern that nursing and midwifery management was preoccupied with hierarchies and the detailed control of nurses and midwives rather than the management of the nursing and midwifery function;

(v)   the need to examine the recruitment, selection and training of nurse/midwife managers in order to ensure that the profession had an effective cohort of leaders capable of responding to changing service needs; and

(vi) the need for the greater devolution of authority within the nursing and midwifery management structure.

Recent Initiatives

7.4 A range of initiatives has taken place recently in relation to the development of management skills within nursing and midwifery. These include a number of master classes organised by the Office for Health Management for directors of nursing and midwifery services of larger acute hospitals and superintendent public health nurses. A nurse management leadership development programme for nurses and midwives under thirty-five years of age is also being provided by the Office for Health Management with the development programme being delivered by a partnership led by the Centre for Nursing Policy and Practice, University of Leeds with the Institute of Public Administration and the Department of Nursing Studies, National University of Ireland - Cork. In addition, the Minister recently announced a major nurse management development programme developed by the Office for Health Management in partnership with the Irish Nurses Organisation and co-funded by the Department of Health and Children and the Irish Nurses Organisation. These programmes are:

- a managing and leading programme for nurse managers from medium sized hospitals provided by the King's Fund;

- a programme for nurse managers from smaller hospitals provided by the University of Limerick;

- a pilot staff/management development programme for all the nursing staff in Longford-Westmeath General Hospital provided by the University of Leeds; and

- a public health nursing leadership programme focused on two neighbouring health boards provided by the Royal College of Nursing.

Internal Communications

7.5 As outlined above, a common concern expressed by nurses and midwives during the consultative process was that they were not informed of decisions or developments within the health service and were given little opportunity to express their views on developments. The communication process did not appear to be effective in conveying information from management to nurses and midwives and in turn conveying information from nurses and midwives to management. It was acknowledged that in some areas substantial efforts had been made in attempting to communicate with all staff in an organisation. Many organisations issue newsletters outlining developments and decisions on future direction. The Southern Health Board, for example, commenced a strategic change programme in 1993 with an increased emphasis on communication. The Commission also understands that a number of organisations have employed management consultants to assist them in developing a communication strategy.

7.6 An effective internal communication system within any organisation is difficult to develop and maintain. Health service providers have the difficulty of communicating with a twenty-four hour nursing and midwifery service. In the case of health boards, the nursing and midwifery service is located in a number of disparate sites. In addition, the different disciplines of nursing may have specific concerns and requirements and health boards must tailor a communication system to be responsive to these divergent needs.

7.7 Nurses and midwives represent a well educated and committed element of the health service. It is essential that health service providers involve nurses and midwives in the development of corporate strategies through programmes of internal communication which build commitment and draw on the full capability of the nursing and midwifery personnel resource. The emphasis should be on a three way process of communication involving management, the nursing organisations and nurses and midwives. The objective should be to create a sense of unifying purpose amongst nurses and midwives and a sense of belonging to an organisation.

7.8   There appears to be a culture in certain areas of the health service of retaining information. It appears that the retention of information is considered as underpinning a command and control model of management. In the absence of the disclosure of information, nurses and midwives will not be able to effectively contribute to the decision making process. There needs to be a culture within health service providers which encourages the full disclosure of information. Managers need to foster an open system of management where information, in relation to service developments and plans, is discussed openly and frankly with nurses and midwives involved in the delivery of services. It was suggested during the consultative process, for example, that many nurse and midwife managers were unaware of the full budget for in-service nurse and midwife training. This in turn lead to suspicions that such funds were diverted to other areas of the health service, which might not in fact have been the case. The greater dissemination of information and a culture within a health service provider which encourages and supports an open flow of information is essential to an effective communications system.

7.9   It is considered that in any communications strategy, the most important source of information to front line staff, is not senior management but their immediate supervisors. An effective communication system requires all levels of management to communicate with the personnel in an immediate reporting relationship. It will be necessary to train, encourage and support all levels of management in communications. It is not sufficient merely to designate a manager as being responsible for communication within an organisation. Effective communication is an essential component of every manager's job. Whilst an organisation can put in place paper and electronic communication systems, the primary and most effective means of communication will remain oral communication at all levels of an organisation. Managers should receive the necessary training to develop their oral communication skills.

7.10   A communication system is not merely about conveying the management perspective to staff but is also about being open to the receipt of information from staff. Management must not only have the capacity to convey information but must also show an equal willingness to listen to and seek the views of nurses and midwives involved in the delivery of services. In the absence of a culture where there is two-way communication (in both directions from management to employees and vice versa), any communication system will be seen merely as a means of conveying management "propaganda". The full utilisation of a well educated and committed workforce means that their views in the planning and delivery of services must be actively sought and mechanisms must be in place to allow an effective input from nurses and midwives. An effective organisation is usually a "listening and learning" organisation.

7.11   An effective communications system also means having open communication with the nursing trade unions. The unions represent nurses and midwives across a wide spectrum of the health services. Management and unions can work in partnership to ensure an effective service which is delivered by an informed and committed workforce. However, an effective communication system with trade unions does not mean management can abrogate its responsibility to communicate directly with nurses and midwives.

7.12   ***The Commission recommends that all health service providers put in place mechanisms for ensuring an effective internal communications system with nurses and midwives. Such systems should be audited on an on-going basis to ensure their continuing effectiveness in conveying and receiving information.***

Professional and Personal Career Planning

7.13   In any workforce and particularly in a professional workforce, there is a need for individuals to develop personal career plans which reflect their abilities and interests. Each nurse or midwife may have particular interests in either clinical practice, education or management and may wish to pursue particular career avenues. There is a need to develop systems which facilitate the desired personal career choices of individual nurses and midwives in the context of the needs of health service providers in meeting organisational and service goals. Developing a personal career plan which will involve identifying the skills, training and educational characteristics and needs of individuals is a challenging process. Such a process involves a real commitment from both management and staff and also requires an understanding from both parties of the purpose and objectives of personal career planning and development. The purpose is to facilitate the development of individuals and is not related to either incremental pay or the disciplinary process. The process is a partnership between employers and staff in developing personal career plans within the context of organisational and service needs. The principles which might underpin personal development planning were recently outlined by Robin Douglas in an article for the Office for Health Management (Office for Health Management: Issue 3, May 1998).

These included:

- an acceptance of personal responsibility for one's own learning;

- a recognition that self knowledge is crucial to effective development;

- an understanding of the many formal and informal opportunities that may be taken to improve knowledge and skills;

- a belief that action-based learning can provide the means to embed substantive knowledge and give the chance to apply ideas to practice;

- the understanding that the process of learning is not a simple change from incompetence to full capability, but contains many challenges in both intellect and emotion that must be met along the way. In other words, to learn, it is often important to unlearn, and for a period perhaps it is necessary to become less competent; and

- an acceptance that, although the responsibility for planning and implementing a personal development plan is likely to be an individual process, work with others will be crucial in achieving any development goals.

7.14   ***The Commission recommends that health service providers introduce systems to facilitate the development of personal career planning amongst nurses and midwives.*** Health service providers should provide training, resources, access to learning opportunities and funding or support for nurses and midwives to acquire new skills and capabilities. Training should be provided to managers and staff in the aims and objectives of personal career planning. Prior to the introduction of any system to facilitate the introduction of a professional and personal career planning system for nurses and midwives, there should be discussions between health service employers and nursing organisations.

The Strategic Planning of the Nursing and Midwifery Service

7.15   The consultative process identified a concern that nurses and midwives did not have an effective input in planning or in policy and strategy development. It was also suggested that there was a need to examine structures of ensuring the more effective development and planning of nursing and midwifery services at health board level. Nursing and midwifery are going through a period of rapid change impacting on the traditional career pathways of nurses and midwives, the parameters of nursing and midwifery practice and the organisation and delivery of nursing and midwifery services. The rapid development of nursing and midwifery, the increasing opportunities for nurses and midwives to focus and specialise in their practice, raises concerns in relation to the potential for increased fragmentation of the nursing and midwifery service. These developments will require the effective planning of the nursing and midwifery resource, particularly in identifying the educational and skills requirement of nursing and midwifery within a health board area.

The Chief Nursing Officer at the Department of Health and Children

7.16   A Chief Nursing Officer was appointed in 1998 to the Department of Health and Children to strengthen its nursing and midwifery policy and planning function. This is a recent appointment and the function is still in the process of development. However, the Commission envisages that the Chief Nursing Officer and her office will have a crucial role in strengthening the central planning and strategic development of nursing and midwifery and in the implementation of the recommendations of this report. There is a need to strengthen the workforce planning, professional leadership and quality assurance functions in the Department of Health and Children. *The Commission recommends the development of the post of Chief Nursing Officer at the Department of Health and Children. The post should be filled on a fixed-term contract basis. Given the crucial role of the post, the Commission recommends that the Chief Nursing Officer be supported by the recruitment of nurses and midwives from the health services.* These nurses and midwives would provide additional professional expertise not readily available within the Department of Health and Children. Such staff should be recruited for up to two year periods from within the health service. Staff could then return to health service providers thus allowing any additional skills or perspectives acquired to be used to the benefit of health service providers whilst allowing a rotation of perspectives and skills into the Department of Health and Children.

A Nursing and Midwifery Planning and Development Unit

7.17   *The Commission recommends the establishment of a Nursing and Midwifery Planning and Development Unit in each health board.* These units would have a strategic planning and policy development role for nursing and midwifery services in a health board area. *The Commission recommends the Nursing and Midwifery Planning and Development Unit have the following general functions:*

- *strategic planning and quality assurance of nursing and midwifery services in a health board area;*

- *co-ordinating the delivery of nursing and midwifery services and improving co-operation between health board and voluntary bodies in the delivery of nursing and midwifery services;*

- *working in partnership with the Chief Nursing Officer in the Department of Health and Children in planning and policy development on nursing and midwifery issues;*

- *overseeing the detailed provision of continuing nursing and midwifery education within a health board area;*

- *liaising with centres of nursing education of health service providers;*

- *developing, monitoring and reviewing the co-ordination and development of multi-disciplinary nursing services within a community care area;*

- *identifying inter-nursing disciplinary and inter-agency training needs and promoting the development of an inter-nursing disciplinary and inter-agency training strategy;*

- *reviewing significant issues in relation to inter-nursing disciplinary and inter-agency co-operation arising from the handling of selected cases; and*

- *assisting in improving internal communications with nurses and midwives in a health board area.*

7.18   **The Commission recommends that the Nursing and Midwifery Planning and Development Unit at health board level be headed by a senior nurse on a fixed-term contract - the Director of the Nursing and Midwifery Planning and Development Unit - who would report to the Chief Executive Officer of a health board.** It is stressed that the Director of the Nursing and Midwifery Planning and Development Unit will not have a direct reporting responsibility for senior nurse and midwife managers in individual institutions but will operate at a strategic planning level in a manner similar to the Chief Nursing Officer at the Department of Health and Children. **The post of Director of the Nursing and Midwifery Planning and Development Unit should be filled by interview following an open competition.** The Nursing and Midwifery Planning and Development Units will require a range of other nursing and midwifery personnel in fulfilling its functions. **The Commission recommends that the nursing and midwifery staff of the Nursing and Midwifery Planning and Development Units be recruited from nursing and midwifery staff within a health board area for periods of up to two years.** This will allow for a greater exposure of nurses and midwives to the planning and policy development function within health boards and will also allow the Nursing and Midwifery Planning and Development Units make greater use of the nursing and midwifery personnel resource within a health board. The rotation of staff within the Nursing and Midwifery Planning and Development Unit should strengthen the operation of the unit and also assist in the development of the nursing and midwifery management function throughout a health board.

Senior Nursing and Midwifery Management

7.19   As previously outlined there was a view expressed that senior nursing and midwifery management concentrated on the individual management of nurses and midwives rather than the management of nursing and midwifery. It was suggested that senior nursing and midwifery management focused on such issues as the rostering of nurses and midwives, sick leave and annual leave rather than the development of nursing and midwifery practice and policies for the more effective delivery of nursing and midwifery care. It was suggested that senior nursing and midwifery management operated on the basis of command and control rather than consultation and the delegation of responsibility.

7.20   The Commission considers that nursing and midwifery require strong professional leadership which can be provided by directors of nursing or chief nursing officers. The strategic planning and professional leadership of nursing and midwifery means that senior nursing and midwifery management cannot be involved in the minutiae of the day to day management of nurses and midwives (such as rostering). The involvement of senior nursing and midwifery management in detailed management issues would also undermine all levels of nursing and midwifery management. In such a scenario other levels of nursing and midwifery management will merely act as "gatekeepers" or "message carriers" for senior nursing and midwifery management. **The Commission recommends that the responsibilities of senior nursing and midwifery management should include:**

- *providing strategic and clinical leadership and direction for nursing and midwifery and related services which results in the delivery of effective, efficient, quality assured and patient centred nursing and midwifery care;*

- *developing a shared sense of commitment and participation amongst staff in the management of change, the development of nursing and midwifery services and in responding to the changing health needs of patients;*

- *developing the concept of care planning in collaboration with other professionals;*

- *participating in the overall financial planning of the health service provided including the assessment of priorities in pay and non-pay expenditure;*

- *ensuring that appropriate in-service education programmes and on-going learning needs are met for all assigned staff; and*

- *ensuring that modern standards of clinical nursing and midwifery care are in operation and that regular monitoring of nursing and midwifery care is undertaken through audit.*

7.21   It is essential that senior nursing and midwifery management empowers all levels of nursing and midwifery in the management and delivery of services. Senior nursing and midwifery management has a crucial role in providing professional leadership to nurses and midwives. This role will be particularly important where there is increased specialisation and the potential for increased fragmentation in the nursing and midwifery service. Senior nursing and midwifery management must ensure continued coherence in the planning and development of nursing and midwifery services.

7.22   In recognition of the increased focus of senior nursing management on the strategic planning of nursing and midwifery services, **the Commission recommends that in future all matrons in large acute hospitals and chief nursing officers in the psychiatric services should be entitled Directors of Nursing**.

Nursing Management in Smaller Hospitals

7.23   The Commission recognises that matrons of smaller hospitals (bands three, four and five) need to combine a professional leadership role with detailed general management responsibilities. Their professional leadership role is just as important as in the larger hospitals, the difference being a matter of scale. They have a crucial role in overseeing the professional development of nurses in their hospitals. It was reported during the consultative process that many such matrons were not involved in the budgetary process. **In order to discharge their general management functions more effectively, the Commission recommends that matrons of smaller hospitals (bands three, four and five) should be given more explicit input into the determination of the budget and greater control and responsibility over its utilisation.** Where savings are achieved, they should be utilised to improve the standard of care or quality of life of the patients.

Middle Nursing and Midwifery Management

7.24   There are numerous titles ascribed to middle nurse and midwife managers in Irish hospitals as outlined in the literature review conducted by Maureen Flynn, on behalf of the Commission.

Examples of these include:

- Night Superintendent;

- Assistant Director of Nursing;

- Assistant Chief Nursing Officer;

- Unit/Divisional Nurse Manager;

- Directorate Nurse Manager;

- Superintendents; and

- Assistant Matrons.

7.25 The roles of nurses and midwives employed in these posts were identified as varying considerably and were described as being generally more administrative than managerial. This has often resulted in confusion amongst staff in relation to those who have responsibility for decision making in areas such as; working arrangements, skill mix, educational requirements or career plans. It appears that in many cases, decisions on these matters are referred to the Director of Nursing or Chief Nursing Officer for decision, with middle nursing and midwifery management merely acting as conduits for information or "gatekeepers". Role conflict, ambiguity and incongruity, if allowed to continue, will undermine the rationale for the continued existence of a layer of middle nursing and midwifery management. There is a need when appointing nurses and midwives to such posts that they be furnished with realistic, explicit and detailed job descriptions and receive the requisite support from senior management. The introduction of new management structures in some services in recent years has meant in many cases that the middle nurse and midwife manager has a clear role and has direct managerial responsibility, authority and accountability for all nurses and midwives in her or his designated area.

7.26 It is essential that middle nursing and midwifery managers have a clearly defined management role, in structures within the health services. In the absence of any clearly defined role such posts may merely carry out a range of administrative duties which may bear little relationship to professional nursing or midwifery. In line with management developments in general, there are increasing calls to replace traditional hierarchical and bureaucratic models of management with flatter structures which empower those at the front line of service delivery. Middle nursing and midwifery management must have its management role clearly defined in the interests of the delivery of more effective, quality patient care.

7.27 The developments of clinical directorates and psychiatric care sectors within the Irish health service in recent years, have helped to provide middle nursing and midwifery management with more clearly defined management roles. Clinical directorates operate in a small number of hospitals as pilot sites at present. Directorates, headed by a clinical director, operate on a triumvirate system of management involving a medical consultant, nurse manager and a business manager. Overall responsibility for the budget and management of clinical services rests with the Clinical Director. Nursing and midwifery managers in this system have devolved authority in relation to the leadership and development of nursing and midwifery personnel within the directorate. In a directorate model, it is essential that nursing and midwifery retain a strong sense of identity and the nursing manager is responsible for ensuring this sense of identity and maintaining the highest standards of professional care for patients. To date, the Clinical Director in all cases is a medical consultant. The current contract for consultants working in the Irish public health service provides that all clinical director posts within clinical directorates should be held by a medical consultant. The Commission has learned from contacts with the United Kingdom and on its visit to Australia that, on occasions, the clinical director post is held by a nurse or midwife in these countries. Such posts are held with the approval of all staff working within a directorate and appear to operate very successfully where a nurse or midwife has a combination of clinical awareness and management skills to manage a directorate effectively. Nurses and midwives may also be in a position to devote their full energies to this crucial function, whilst often medical consultants have little time to devote to their management responsibilities because of time demands in the treatment of public and private patients. In discussions with representatives of the Irish Hospital Consultants Association, it was stated that they would have no objection to a nurse or midwife being clinical director of a directorate where this was agreed with the clinical team. **The Commission recommends that consideration should be given to the appointment of nurse or midwife managers as clinical directors, where appropriate.**

7.28 In hospitals where clinical directorates have not been introduced, middle nursing and midwifery management has also worked effectively in taking on explicit functional roles or in the management of areas of care (such as surgical units of care). The functional roles have included bed management and practice development co-ordination. The Commission learned during its visit to Australia of middle nursing and midwifery management taking on roles in relation to the management of housekeeping and catering services, the co-ordination of nursing and midwifery services across a range of care areas and the nursing and midwifery research and continuing education function within a hospital.

7.29 *The Commission recommends that middle nursing and midwifery management should:*

- *have a defined management role and not merely retain a "gatekeeping" administrative function;*

- *have defined management responsibility with explicit delegation of authority from directors of nursing and chief nursing officers;*

- *have definite functional roles either in managing units of care or in the management of functional responsibilities such as in bed management and practice development co-ordination; and*

- *have the authority to manage their area of responsibility without constant reference to more senior management. However, as in all management, there should be effective communication with front-line and senior management.*

7.30 The Commission also considers that there should be a greater nursing and midwifery management input in areas which impact directly on the quality of care. These areas include catering, cleaning and laundry services. The Commission considers that nursing management should be involved in discussions on the award of contracts for such services.

First Line Nursing and Midwifery Management

7.31 The role of the ward sister and nursing officer (first line nursing managers) was widely acknowledged throughout the consultative fora and in written submissions as being crucial to the effective running of the hospital or service - ward sisters and nursing officers were often described as the "lynchpin". However, in the literature review undertaken by Maureen Flynn on behalf of the Commission it was found that there are large variances in the levels of autonomy and control given to first line managers across hospitals in Ireland.

7.32 Traditionally, staff nurses/midwives, in the absence of a clinical career pathway, have been promoted to ward sister and nursing officer on the basis of their competence and experience in the clinical field. However, good clinical nurses or midwives have not always made good nurse and midwife managers and this has been compounded by the fact that in many places ward sisters continue to be rostered in the staffing complement with a patient caseload, to the detriment of managing the ward. While clinical credibility is seen to be intrinsic to the role, the amount of time that a ward sister or nursing officer can devote to clinical practice varies considerably, depending on whether he or she is employed in a small district or a large tertiary health care facility.

7.33 Changes in the health services, such as much shorter lengths of stay in hospital, the increasingly acute nature of patients in hospital and the ever rapid rate of technological development have all impacted on the role of first line nursing and midwifery managers across the health service. The management of care in nursing and midwifery increasingly calls for a range of well developed personnel and resource management skills in the ward sister and nursing officer. In many instances, first line nursing managers have not received appropriate management training or upskilling for their role as it has evolved in recent years. Many first line nursing and midwifery managers appear to have undertaken courses on their own initiative without acquiring management skills appropriate for the effective discharge of their duties.

7.34   First line nursing and midwifery managers need not only to develop management skills, but also retain the need to act as professional leaders amongst nurses and midwives working on a ward or in a service area by maintaining clinical credibility. The key nature of the management and professional leadership role of first line nursing and midwifery managers was identified by Lewis in 1990 in a study which suggests that:

- first line nursing and midwifery managers exert such influence that they have the potential to effectively negate any changes in the professional function and therefore should be involved in all discussions in relation to change;

- in order to control the nursing and midwifery function effectively, first line nursing and midwifery managers should be expert in the three processes of the nursing and midwifery function; defining, managing and practising. First line nursing and midwifery managers must therefore have further education in theory relating to nursing and midwifery frameworks, management and practice; and

- as the maintenance of high professional standards is essential to the public interest, the clinical function of their role must not be sublimated to the managerial function.

7.35   In 1994, a review of twenty years of literature from both the USA and the UK regarding supportive supervision and the role of the nurse manager/ward sister was published. The research from both countries found that all nurses and midwives from student nurse to middle manager are seeking in their supervisor a person who will *"enable them to give of their best while obtaining satisfaction from their work, rather than a controlling supervisor who attempts to mould them into a group of subservient drones"* (Cameron Buccheri and Ogier, 1994). The authors suggest that the behaviour of supportive supervisors includes: demonstrating value for nurses and midwives as individuals; recognising their worth; allowing them to express their opinions and assisting them in decision making and problem solving by communicating adequate information. The authors offer four basic suggestions for supporting first line nurse and midwife managers in their role:

- they must be given adequate resources to develop their expertise as health resource managers;

- they should be given frequent feedback in relation to their own performance;

- too much emphasis should not be placed on the managerial functions of the first line nursing and midwifery manager at the expense of the clinical aspects of their role; and

- first line nursing and midwifery managers should have support from middle and senior management by sharing information with them, encouraging them to have an influence on their organisation and its policies and by assisting them to receive recognition within the organisation.

7.36   The combination of managerial functions and clinical/professional leadership required of first line nursing and midwifery managers calls for a significant level of managerial competence together with clinical credibility. The combination of both these functions needs to be carefully managed and supported by senior management. A ward sister or nursing officer should receive adequate support to ensure that both functions are effectively performed in the interest of the delivery of an efficient, effective and high quality health service. ***The Commission recommends that clerical and information technology support be made available to first line nursing and midwifery managers to support them in their managerial function, where appropriate.***

7.37   In order to manage effectively the delivery of health care on a ward or in a service area and promote high standards of care, the control of resources should be delegated to the ward or unit of service delivery. The Audit Commission, in the United Kingdom, published a document entitled - *Making Time for Patients* - in 1992 which examined the role of ward sisters in the National Health Service. The report identified problems attaching to the split between responsibility for the ward and control over resources. Historically, responsibility for ward resources and the clinical activity on the ward has tended to be split between the managers above and outside the ward who control the resources and the ward sister who is responsible for patient care. The report advocates decentralised management structures that bring the two more closely together. A recent economic review of the Irish health services found that:

*"the management of the hospital system seems to be unduly centralised and bureaucratic…
Moreover, in a hospital it is rare for budget responsibility to be devolved to operating units" (OECD, 1997)*

7.38   The Commission supports the view that, in line with the Health Strategy - *Shaping a Healthier Future* - budgets should be devolved to the units of service delivery. It is recognised that the management information and support systems used by many health service providers will not support the effective devolution of budgetary responsibility. **The Commission recommends investment in the management information and support systems used by health service providers to allow for greater devolution of budgetary responsibility which would result in significant improvements in the effective and efficient utilisation of resources.**

7.39   **The Commission recommends that first line nursing and midwifery management should be given greater budgetary responsibility in relation to the utilisation of resources at units of service delivery.** It is an essential ingredient of functional management to be involved in controlling, preparing and monitoring the budget. Front line nursing and midwifery management should have this responsibility and be supported in developing the necessary skills to perform this function effectively. It is essential that first line nursing and midwifery management receive training in analysing, constructing and monitoring budgets. It is acknowledged that currently many factors which will impinge on resource utilisation at the unit of service delivery may be outside the control of first line nursing and midwifery management; these factors include for example the ordering of excessive clinical tests by junior medical staff, the admission and discharge of patients and the requirement of one to one nursing ("specialling") ordered by a medical consultant. The effective management of resources at units of service delivery requires a partnership between all professionals involved in the delivery of services to clients and patients, particularly between nurses/midwives and medical professionals. The elements of the budget to be controlled by first line nursing and midwifery management should be agreed by all those involved in care teams, but should include at a minimum nursing/midwifery and ancillary staff pay costs and supplies. If savings are made, it should be clear to what extent such savings can be utilised within the ward.

7.40   The Commission recognises that these proposals involve a significant increase in the management responsibilities currently expected of many first line nursing and midwifery managers and must be balanced with maintaining effective clinical and professional leadership. Prior to the devolution of additional budgetary and management responsibilities, those who currently hold first line management positions must be supported in developing their skills. The Office for Health Management should identify the range of skills required by first line nursing and midwifery management to perform a clinical leadership and a resource and personnel management function. **The Commission recommends that training programmes should be organised in partnership between health boards, voluntary agencies and the Office for Health Management to develop and support existing first line nursing and midwifery managers to enable them to take on additional management and budgetary responsibilities.**

7.41   Front line nursing and midwifery managers have an enormous impact on the culture of care in a hospital or service with a resulting impact on the quality of patient care. It is essential that ward sisters and nursing officers are seen as a key management grade within the health service whilst at the same time retaining a clinical and professional leadership role. **The Commission recommends the development of first line nursing and midwifery management to fulfil the following functions:**

- *professional/clinical leadership;*

- *staffing and staff development;*

- *resource management; and*

- *facilitating communication.*

The Commission also recommends that first line nursing and midwifery managers should have management training before taking up a post and be required and supported in continuing to develop management skills. The development of management skills should operate in tandem with maintaining clinical credibility by being aware of changes in clinical practice.

7.42   The title of ward sister may be regarded as an anachronism in the modern health service and it has been suggested that the function might be more appropriately titled "Clinical Nurse Manager" or "Clinical Midwife Manager". This title may more adequately reflect what the Commission envisages as the key functions of first line nursing and midwifery management; resource management, staffing and staff development, facilitating communication and professional/clinical leadership. This title might also be considered by the psychiatric nursing services. The ward sister would be entitled Clinical Nurse Manager 2 or Clinical Midwife Manager 2.

7.43   The post of junior ward sister has been alternatively described as a useful preparation for nursing and midwifery management and as a "non-job" merely acting as an aid to a ward sister. The Commission is aware that the post of junior ward sister was used in some cases as an alternative to a ward sister post, which should not happen. The Commission having considered the matter was of the view that there was a need for an additional post in the management of a ward, where required by the activity and complexity of the nursing/midwifery service, below the ward sister or nursing officer. A person filling such a post should have a clearly defined role and responsibility and would normally take charge in the absence of a ward sister or nursing officer. The junior ward sister would in all cases report to the ward sister in her/his area. In the psychiatric services there is at least one deputy nursing officer in most units of care. The post of deputy nursing officer is similar but not identical to junior ward sister. This post would be entitled Clinical Nurse Manager 1 or Clinical Midwife Manager 1.

7.44   There is also the need for a level of first line nursing and midwifery management above that of ward sister and nursing officer in areas where it is justified by the complexity and level of activity. The Commission envisages that it will be extremely rare for all three levels of nursing and midwifery management to be in the same unit. However, in an area such as Accident and Emergency in a large tertiary acute hospital there may be a requirement for a number of ward sisters and the Commission considers that one person should be designated as being in charge of the unit. It is in such a scenario that the Commission envisages a level of first line nursing and midwifery management above that of ward sister. The other ward sisters would report to this higher level of first line nursing and midwifery management. The post would be entitled Clinical Nurse Manager 3 or Clinical Midwife Manager 3.

7.45   **In summary the Commission recommends that there should be three grades of first line nursing and midwifery management in the health service.** All three grades would rarely be in place in a single unit and only one person would be designated as being in overall charge of a single unit of care or ward. *The Commission recommends that the title used for first line nursing and midwifery management be "Clinical Nurse Manager" or "Clinical Midwife Manager". The three grades would be:*

- *Clinical Nurse Manager 1 or Clinical Midwife Manager 1 (reporting to a Clinical Nurse or Midwife Manger 2);*

- *Clinical Nurse Manager 2 or Clinical Midwife Manager 2 (in charge of a ward or unit of care); and*

- *Clinical Nurse Manager 3 or Clinical Midwife Manager 3 (in charge of a department).*

The three first line nursing and midwifery management grades would reflect the three levels of first line nursing and midwifery management referred to in this section. *The conditions of employment of these posts should be determined in the appropriate fora.*

Promotion and Related Difficulties

7.46   It is important that the most suitable nurses are attracted into management. This will not happen if financial and other rewards are not in place. The issue of differentials between the staff nurse and ward sister/nursing officer grades has been the subject of concern and dispute since the early 1970's when premium pay was introduced in response to a request by nurses working unsocial hours. Since then, national wage agreements and grade increases have failed to resolve the problem which has been exacerbated by the last pay award to nurses.

7.47   The Commission considers that existing differentials constitute the main difficulty relating to promotion. Current pay structures seriously mitigate against encouraging nurses to avail of promotional opportunities. The loss of premium earnings frequently means that the ward sister/nursing officer in a promotional position earns less than a staff nurse. This makes it financially unattractive for nurses at present to seek promotion into the more senior nursing posts where premium payments do not apply. Many hospital/agencies find it difficult to encourage nurses to seek promotion.

7.48   The problems related to promotion are not just emphasised by nurses but are also recognised by the chief executive officers of the health boards and voluntary hospitals in their submissions.

7.49   Another factor which must be taken into account in relation to promotion is that unlike almost every other occupation in the health services, nursing does not have a system of incremental leave. A director of nursing gets the same number of annual days leave as a staff nurse.

7.50   *The Commission recommends that differentials and incremental annual leave in promotional grades be examined as a matter of urgency, before the end of December 1998, through the established structures. To this examination should be added the effect of the enhanced role for ward sisters and higher grades which has been recommended by the Commission earlier in this chapter.*

Nurses and Midwives in General Management

7.51   As stated previously nursing and midwifery provide a valuable personnel resource to the health services. Nurses and midwives have an in-depth knowledge of the health services and are particularly aware of the needs of patients and clients of the health services. Nurses and midwives possess a range of clinical skills and awareness which, if combined with management expertise, offer a potentially valuable management recruitment pool. The Commission was concerned that nurses and midwives in pursuing management roles in the health service appear to focus almost exclusively on roles within nursing and midwifery management. The Commission considers that nurses and midwives should seek opportunities in general management. The exposure of nurses and midwives to a wider range of management responsibilities would benefit both general management and nursing and midwifery. The nursing and midwifery perspective and awareness of clinical issues would be an invaluable attribute in a general management role. Similarly the exposure of nurses and midwives to wider general health service issues would benefit nursing and midwifery management should a nurse or midwife return to nursing and midwifery management at a later stage. *The Commission recommends that health service providers encourage nurses and midwives to seek opportunities in general management and that nurses and midwives consider pursuing careers in general health service management.*

Recruitment and Selection of Nurse and Midwife Managers

7.52 The recruitment and selection process for nurse and midwife managers was considered by the Commission. It was felt that when advertising for a nursing or midwifery management position, the job description should contain a requirement that applicants must have undergone a management course and have adequate experience relevant to the post. *The Commission recommends that the Office for Health Management approve appropriate management courses for each particular level of nursing and midwifery management. The Commission also recommends that nurse and midwife managers at each level in the health service should have an appropriate management qualification and/or experience relevant to the post.*

7.53 *The Commission recommends that the Office for Health Management carry out a survey into the competencies required for nursing and midwifery management positions.* These competencies should be drawn up in the light of the management responsibilities identified for each level of nursing and midwifery management by the Commission.

7.54 The issue of nurse or midwife managers' posts remaining vacant for long periods was raised during the consultative process. Nurse and midwife managers "acting-up" for long periods in management positions was not seen to be in the best interests of effective management but was disempowering and demoralising for all concerned. *The Commission recommends that vacant management posts where nurses or midwives are "acting up" should be filled as soon as possible.*

7.55 When the Commission met with directors of nursing of large acute hospitals in September 1997, they voiced their dissatisfaction in relation to their non-involvement in the recruitment and selection of middle nurse managers for their own hospital, competitions for which are handled by the Local Appointments Commission. They considered it very important that they would be involved in choosing someone who in their opinion would "fit in" with the ethos of the hospital and this would allow for better succession planning. The Commission considered that in the modern health service there may no longer be a requirement for the Local Appointments Commission to be involved in the selection and recruitment of middle nursing and midwifery managers. The selection and recruitment process could be organised by a health board or health service provider itself. *Therefore, the Commission recommends that the Local Appointments Commission should no longer be involved in administering the selection and recruitment of middle nursing and midwifery managers.*

Management Development

7.56 A number of management development programmes have been provided for nurses and midwives by the Office for Health Management as identified in paragraph 7.4. These are welcome initiatives and reflect the need to develop current nursing and midwifery managers and future leaders. Nursing and midwifery, like other areas of the health service, will continue to need to develop and evolve rapidly in response to changing client needs and social circumstances. As outlined already, future nurse and midwife managers will require a range of resource management, communication and personnel skills to ensure the provision of an effective and efficient health service. These skills need to be developed and efforts need to be made to give nurses and midwives opportunities to develop these skills. In particular, nurses and midwives should be encouraged to participate in third-level post graduate management courses.

7.57 The increasing inter-disciplinary nature of the provision of health services requires co-ordination of professional and administrative services. In developing management skills it is important that all groups share ideas and perspectives. ***Therefore, the Commission recommends that, where appropriate, nursing and midwifery management development programmes should be run in conjunction with management programmes for other professional groups and general managers.***

The Personnel Management of Nursing and Midwifery

7.58 The Commission in this chapter has recommended a revised management framework for nursing which refocuses the activities of senior nursing management on a strategic planning and quality assurance role. The management of staff, it is recommended, should be delegated to units of care. The effective management of nursing and midwifery staff is crucial to the delivery of high quality care within the health services. As identified in chapter two on the evolution of the nursing profession in Ireland, the traditional management of nurses and midwives reflected a rigid hierarchical culture derived from a semi-militaristic and religious service background. The consultative process identified a series of issues in relation to the management of nurses and midwives which should be addressed in the context of the revised nursing and midwifery management framework.

The Shortage of Nurses and Midwives

7.59 The Commission is aware that there is currently a shortage of nurses in certain areas of the country. There also appears to be a shortage of nurses for certain specialist areas such as theatre nursing. The shortage emerged during the life of the Commission and whilst not researched in great detail may be due to a variety of factors such as the change in status of nursing students from employee to supernumerary and the on-going well-being of the Irish economy in general which means that there are increased opportunities outside of the health services for nurses. In addressing staff shortages, nursing management needs to be flexible and creative in the working opportunities offered to nurses. Opportunities should be created for those currently working outside of Ireland or not practising nursing to return to the workforce.

Flexible Working Arrangements

7.60 It was suggested during the consultative process that there was a need for greater flexibility in the hours worked by nurses and midwives at different levels. As a predominantly female profession, it was believed that increased access to and availability of job sharing or permanent part-time work ought to be encouraged to allow nurses and midwives combine satisfactorily their professional and family roles. Such flexibility in working arrangements was considered important in order to retain many highly qualified and competent nurses and midwives in the work force, instead of being employed in a temporary capacity.

7.61 Some nurses and midwives also raised the issue of obstacles to transferring either between hospitals in a health board area or between health boards, where a suitable vacancy existed. It was also stated that nurses were not able to move directly to a permanent post but had to take up temporary employment when moving between health boards or some hospitals within the same health board. A further complaint was that having reached a certain increment level whilst employed in one health board they had to revert to the bottom of the incremental scale on taking up temporary employment with another health board.

7.62 ***The Commission recommends that the Health Service Employers Agency and nursing unions develop an agreed framework for the provision of permanent part-time contracts of employment for nurses and midwives.*** The framework should provide for more flexible working opportunities for nurses and midwives and allow for a closer correlation between service need and the personal circumstances of individual nurses. Such permanent part-time contracts might require a nurse or midwife to work a certain number of hours per week or alternatively a specified number of weeks each year which could be concentrated in a period of maximum service need. These permanent part-time contracts should also provide for pension and other entitlements, such as sick leave and maternity leave. ***The Commission recommends that the Health Service Employers Agency and nursing unions examine the equity of current arrangements for nurses and midwives seeking to move from one health board to another or from one hospital to another within a health board.***

The Effective Utilisation of the Professional Skills of Nurses and Midwives

7.63 The interim report of the Commission had identified the concerns of many nurses and midwives at the number of non-nursing or midwifery tasks which they were required to perform. It was suggested that the performance of such tasks did not make best use of the professional nursing and midwifery workforce. ***The Commission*** supports this view and ***recommends that health service providers, nursing and midwifery management and nursing organisations examine opportunities for the increased use of care assistants and other non-nursing personnel in the performance of non-nursing tasks.*** There is also a need to develop mechanisms which will assist in appropriately determining nursing and midwifery staffing levels. A number of such systems may be required, given the variable patient and client dependency, activity levels and the variety of settings in which nurses and midwives work. These mechanisms should also take account of the examination of opportunities for the increased use of care assistants and non-nursing personnel. ***The Commission recommends that the Department of Health and Children, health service providers and nursing organisations examine the development of appropriate systems to determine nursing staffing levels.***

Hand-Over Time

7.64 Another issue identified by nurses and midwives was the fact that in some hospitals hand-over time between shifts was not rostered and the nurses and midwives involved were not paid for this extra time. In other hospitals hand-over time was rostered. ***The Commission recommends that staffing arrangements should be designed to ensure that nurses and midwives are not required to undertake hand-over duties in their own time.***

The Selection and Recruitment of Nurses and Midwives

7.65 The view was expressed during the consultative process that systems for the selection and recruitment of nurses and midwives in certain areas of the health service were overly centralised and bureaucratic. ***The Commission recommends that the systems used for the selection and recruitment of nurses and midwives should be kept under review and should reflect current best practice.***

Temporary Nurses and Midwives

7.66 The consultative process also identified concerns in relation to the number of long-term temporary nurses in the health services. The Commission is aware that health service employers and the nursing unions have agreed that the overall approach to temporary employment should be governed by the principle that the volume of temporary employment in the system should be reduced to the minimum level consistent with operational requirements. Agreement was also reached that 2,000 nursing posts be converted from temporary to whole time permanent status by means of a confined competition. The Commission understands that this process is underway and that over 1,200 temporary nurses and midwives have been appointed to permanent positions since the commencement of the scheme. However, the Commission considers that there may be scope for the process to move at a quicker pace. The Commission is strongly of the view that the level of long-term temporary nurses in the health service, prior to the agreement between employers and unions, seriously impacted on the morale of the profession. This should not be allowed to recur. It is not in the best interests of the provision of a high quality health service that there are large numbers of long-term temporary nursing posts. The Commission strongly supports the agreement between employers and unions that the level of temporary employment in the service be kept to the minimum level consistent with operational requirements. ***The Commission recommends that vacant permanent posts should be filled without delay. A framework should be put in place, following discussions between the Health Service Employers Agency and nursing unions, to ensure the problem does not recur.***

The Quality of the Working Environment

7.67 The issue of compassionate leave for nurses and midwives was also raised during the consultative process. Complaints were made that compassionate leave, which could be for periods of three to five days following bereavement, depending on the circumstances, did not take into account actual rostered time off occurring during the period. The Commission considers that cases should be dealt with on an individual basis. ***The Commission recommends that decisions on compassionate leave be delegated to local management so that there could be greater flexibility in granting additional compassionate leave, in appropriate cases.***

7.68 The issue of the personal security of nurses in the workplace was raised during the consultative process. Many concerns were expressed at what was perceived as the lack of security afforded to nurses in particular situations, for example in the community, isolated hospital settings and emergency departments. Nurses and midwives reported being subjected to both verbal and even physical abuse from clients. Public health nurses reported being exposed to threatening situations either in very isolated areas or in inner-city areas with major socio-economic problems. It was stated that such nurses were very vulnerable as they were not equipped with mobile phones or personal alarms to enable them to call for help. It was submitted that nurses working in isolated settings felt particularly vulnerable at night. Some submissions from psychiatric nurses highlighted the increased exposure of nurses to violent behaviour. The relative isolation of some psychiatric units meant that sometimes there was no immediate back-up in crisis situations.

7.69 The Safety, Health and Welfare at Work Act 1989 (the Health and Safety Act) places a duty of care on every employer to ensure, as far as is reasonably practicable, the safety, health and welfare at work of all employees within an organisation. Therefore there is an obligation on every employer to put in place appropriate safeguards to ensure that the safety of employees within the workplace is protected. Staff also have a role to play in being conscious of the potential abuse and violence in certain circumstances and in taking steps to defuse a potentially hazardous situation. Employers in meeting their obligations under the Health and Safety Act should make use of new technology such as mobile phones or personal alarms. There needs to be investment by employers and consultation with nursing organisations to ensure the personal security of nurses and midwives in the workplace.

7.70   Many health service providers have occupational health programmes providing occupational health support to nurses and midwives. However, such programmes are not uniformly available throughout the health service. ***The Commission recommends the on-going development of occupational health programmes where they are currently provided and their introduction in areas of the health service where they are not currently available.***

7.71   The Sick Doctors Scheme was established primarily to assist doctors who have a substance abuse problem. Referrals are mainly from colleagues but may also come from employing authorities, nurses or occasionally a member of the public. On referral, doctors are assessed and advised on a particular course of treatment - those who require admission to a hospital or centre are liable for their own medical expenses. Financial assistance, by means of an interest free loan over five years, is provided to those who need it. Funding for the scheme is provided through the Irish Medical Organisation (IMO), Irish College of General Practitioners (ICGP), General Practitioner Wives Association and the General Practitioners Benevolent Fund. The scheme is administered by a committee comprising two representatives from each of the following organisations - Irish Medical Organisation and Irish College of General Practitioners. Others may be co-opted as necessary. Anonymity and confidentiality are seen as essential to the successful operation of the scheme. An occupational health programme for doctors is currently being set-up under the auspices of the IMO and the ICGP. Among the services to be provided will be a help-line and counselling.

7.72   The Commission considers that a similar scheme would be beneficial for nurses and midwives. ***The Commission recommends that the nursing unions and other relevant organisations establish a scheme to support nurses and midwives similar to the Sick Doctors Scheme.***

7.73   The issue of a facility for the debriefing of nurses and midwives following critical incidents was also raised during the consultative process. Submissions to the Commission described situations where nurses having dealt with the consequences of a major accident were expected to continue with their work or go off duty without having had the opportunity of discussing the experience with anyone. The Commission is aware that many health service providers have a critical incident debriefing system for nurses and midwives. However, not all nurses and midwives avail of these facilities because of sensitivity that by using such a service there will be an impression that they cannot cope with the job. The culture which prevents nurses and midwives from seeking help when required needs to be addressed by nursing and midwifery management. ***The Commission recommends that where critical incident debriefing systems are not in place they should be developed as a matter of urgency.***

7.74   Many nurses and midwives during the consultative process requested the provision of a professional confidential counselling service. It was suggested that such a service would allow nurses to receive counselling outside of their local environment and away from colleagues with whom they may be required to work subsequently. A number of health boards and voluntary agencies offer a confidential counselling system to their employees. The Commission considers the provision of a confidential counselling system as a vital support to nurses and midwives working in a daily stressful environment. ***The Commission recommends that all health service providers should ensure the availability of a professional confidential counselling system for nurses and midwives in their employment.***

7.75   The question of sick leave for nurses and midwives was also raised during the consultative process. Some nurses and midwives suggested that sick leave incurred as a consequence of an injury at work should be treated as separate from the sick leave scheme. The Commission is of the view that the provision of sick leave is an issue for local nursing and midwifery management and personnel units. ***The Commission recommends that nursing and midwifery management should be enabled to use their discretion to a greater extent to allow for greater flexibility in the*** *provision of sick leave in certain exceptional circumstances.* The Commission has been informed that a scheme is in place which provides for the payment of an allowance (related to salary) to a nurse or midwife, employed by a health board or voluntary hospital, who is absent from work as a result of a serious physical assault incurred in the course of her or his duty. The scheme also covers medical expenses such as those relating to general practitioner or consultant visits or prescription charges. The Commission understands that the scheme will shortly be extended to include nurses working for voluntary mental handicap agencies. *The Commission recommends that details of the scheme be circulated generally.*

7.76 The issue of rest facilities for nurses and midwives was also raised during the consultative process. It was suggested that in many health care facilities there were no, or barely adequate, changing and rest rooms for nurses and midwives. Modern employment practice suggests that staff should have adequate rest facilities on-site and this may be particularly the case in the physically demanding and stressful work environment of nursing and midwifery. *The Commission recommends that health service providers ensure the provision of adequate rest and changing facilities for nurses and midwives.*

7.77 The question was raised during the consultative process of the point of entry on the incremental pay scale of nurses and midwives who had spent a number of years working abroad. It was stated that nurses and midwives returning to Ireland to take up a permanent position in the health service took up employment on the first point of the incremental pay scale. There was a view that such nurses and midwives were a valuable asset to the Irish health service having gained experience and alternative perspectives on care whilst working abroad. The Commission considered the question of the point of entry on the incremental pay scale essentially a matter for local nursing and midwifery management. *The Commission recommends that if a nurse or midwife has acquired skills and experience abroad which are of value to the service, then a nurse or midwife manager should have sufficient discretion within budget to allow her or him to determine the point of entry on the incremental pay scale according to local priorities and needs.*

The Financing of Management Systems

7.78 It will be important to have services in place to support the nursing and midwifery management structures proposed by the Commission. The development of effective management systems and staff development needs to be underpinned by adequate resources. Staff development and management systems should not be seen as a "poor relation" in terms of priorities within the health services. Monies spent on the direct delivery of services will be more effectively utilised if the management structures and staff development programmes are supported by continuing adequate resources and not merely when there is some scope for extra expenditure in the system. *The Commission recommends that there should be long-term financial commitment to developing communication, management information and support systems to allow for greater devolution of budgets and staff development programmes. These programmes need to be underpinned by the allocation of adequate resources and a commitment to on-going funding.*

The Commission recommends that all health service providers put in place mechanisms for ensuring an effective internal communications system with nurses and midwives. Such systems should be audited on an on-going basis to ensure their continuing effectiveness in conveying and receiving information. (7.12)

The Commission recommends that health service providers introduce systems to facilitate the development of personal career planning amongst nurses and midwives. (7.14)

The Commission recommends the development of the post of Chief Nursing Officer at the Department of Health and Children. The post should be filled on a fixed-term contract basis. (7.16)

The Commission recommends that the Chief Nursing Officer be supported by the recruitment of nurses and midwives from the health services. (7.16)

The Commission recommends the establishment of a Nursing and Midwifery Planning and Development Unit in each health board. The Commission recommends the Nursing and Midwifery Planning and Development Unit have the following general functions:

- strategic planning and quality assurance of nursing and midwifery services in a health board area;

- co-ordinating the delivery of nursing and midwifery services and improving co-operation between health board and voluntary bodies in the delivery of nursing and midwifery services;

- working in partnership with the Chief Nursing Officer in the Department of Health and Children in planning and policy development on nursing and midwifery issues;

- overseeing the detailed provision of continuing nursing and midwifery education within a health board area;

- liaising with centres of nursing education of health service providers;

- developing, monitoring and reviewing the co-ordination and development of multi-disciplinary nursing services within a community care area;

- identifying inter-nursing disciplinary and inter-agency training needs and promoting the development of an inter-nursing disciplinary and inter-agency training strategy;

- reviewing significant issues in relation to inter-nursing disciplinary and inter-agency co-operation arising from the handling of selected cases; and

- assisting in improving internal communications with nurses and midwives in a health board area. (7.17)

The Commission recommends that the Nursing and Midwifery Planning and Development Unit at health board level be headed by a senior nurse on a fixed-term contract - the Director of the Nursing and Midwifery Planning and Development Unit - who would report to the Chief Executive Officer of a health board. The post of Director of the Nursing and Midwifery Planning and Development Unit should be filled by interview following an open competition. (7.18)

The Commission recommends that the nursing and midwifery staff of the Nursing and Midwifery Planning and Development Units be recruited from nursing and midwifery staff within a health board area for periods of up to two years. (7.18)

The Commission recommends that the responsibilities of senior nursing and midwifery management should include:

- providing strategic and clinical leadership and direction for nursing and midwifery and related services which results in the delivery of effective, efficient, quality assured and patient centred nursing and midwifery care;

- developing a shared sense of commitment and participation amongst staff in the management of change, the development of nursing and midwifery services and in responding to the changing health needs of patients;

- developing the concept of care planning in collaboration with other professionals;

- participating in the overall financial planning of the health service provided including the assessment of priorities in pay and non-pay expenditure;

- ensuring that appropriate in-service education programmes and on-going learning needs are met for all assigned staff; and

- ensuring that modern standards of clinical nursing and midwifery care are in operation and that regular monitoring of nursing and midwifery care is undertaken through audit. (7.20)

The Commission recommends that in future all matrons in large acute hospitals and chief nursing officers in the psychiatric services should be entitled Directors of Nursing. (7.22)

In order to discharge their general management functions more effectively, the Commission recommends that matrons of smaller hospitals (bands three, four and five) should be given more explicit input into the determination of the budget and greater control and responsibility over its utilisation. (7.23)

The Commission recommends that consideration should be given to the appointment of nurse or midwife managers as clinical directors, where appropriate. (7.27)

The Commission recommends that middle nursing and midwifery management should:

- have a defined management role and not merely retain a "gatekeeping" administrative function;

- have defined management responsibility with explicit delegation of authority from directors of nursing and chief nursing officers;

- have definite functional roles either in managing units of care or in the management of functional responsibilities such as in bed management and practice development co-ordination; and

- have the authority to manage their area of responsibility without constant reference to more senior management. However, as in all management, there should be effective communication with front-line and senior management. (7.29)

The Commission recommends that clerical and information technology support be made available to first line nursing and midwifery managers to support them in their managerial function, where appropriate. (7.36)

The Commission recommends investment in the management information and support systems used by health service providers to allow for greater devolution of budgetary responsibility, which would result in significant improvements in the effective and efficient utilisation of resources. (7.38)

The Commission recommends that first line nursing and midwifery management should be given greater budgetary responsibility in relation to the utilisation of resources at units of service delivery. (7.39)

The Commission recommends that training programmes should be organised in partnership between health boards, voluntary organisations and the Office for Health Management to develop and support existing first line nursing and midwifery managers to enable them to take on additional management and budgetary responsibilities. (7.40)

The Commission recommends the development of first line nursing and midwifery management to fulfil the following functions:

- professional/clinical leadership;

- staffing and staff development;

- resource management; and

- facilitating communication. (7.41)

The Commission recommends that first line nursing and midwifery managers should have management training before taking up a post and be required and supported in continuing to develop management skills. The development of management skills should operate in tandem with maintaining clinical credibility by being aware of changes in clinical practice. (7.41)

The Commission recommends that there should be three grades of first line nursing and midwifery management in the health service. The Commission recommends that the title used for first line nursing and midwifery management be "Clinical Nurse Manager" or "Clinical Midwife Manager". The three grades would be:

- Clinical Nurse Manager 1 or Clinical Midwife Manager 1 (reporting to a Clinical Nurse or Midwife Manager 2);

- Clinical Nurse Manager 2 or Clinical Midwife Manager 2 (in charge of a ward or unit of care); and

- Clinical Nurse Manager 3 or Clinical Midwife Manager 3 (in charge of a department).

The conditions of employment of these posts should be determined in the appropriate fora. (7.45)

The Commission recommends that differentials and incremental annual leave in promotional grades be examined as a matter of urgency, before the end of December 1998, through the established structures. To this examination should be added the effect of the enhanced role for ward sisters and higher grades which has been recommended by the Commission. (7.50)

The Commission recommends that health service providers encourage nurses and midwives to seek opportunities in general management and that nurses and midwives consider pursuing careers in general health service management. (7.51)

The Commission recommends that the Office for Health Management approve appropriate management courses for each particular level of nursing and midwifery management. The Commission also recommends that nurse and midwife managers at each level in the health service should have an appropriate management qualification and/or experience relevant to the post. (7.52)

The Commission recommends that the Office for Health Management carry out a survey into the competencies required for nursing and midwifery management positions. (7.53)

The Commission recommends that vacant management posts where nurses or midwives are "acting-up" should be filled as soon as possible. (7.54)

The Commission recommends that the Local Appointments Commission should no longer be involved in administering the selection and recruitment of middle nursing and midwifery managers. (7.55)

The Commission recommends that, where appropriate, nursing and midwifery management development programmes should be run in conjunction with management programmes for other professional groups and general managers. (7.57)

The Commission recommends that the Health Service Employers Agency and nursing unions develop an agreed framework for the provision of permanent part-time contracts of employment for nurses and midwives. (7.62)

The Commission recommends that the Health Service Employers Agency and nursing unions examine the equity of current arrangements for nurses and midwives seeking to move from one health board to another or from one hospital to another within a health board. (7.62)

The Commission recommends that health service providers, nursing and midwifery management and nursing organisations examine opportunities for the increased use of care assistants and other non-nursing personnel in the performance of non-nursing tasks. (7.63)

The Commission recommends that the Department of Health and Children, health service providers and nursing organisations examine the development of appropriate systems to determine nursing staffing levels. (7.63)

The Commission recommends that staffing arrangements should be designed to ensure that nurses and midwives are not required to undertake hand-over duties in their own time. (7.64)

The Commission recommends that the systems used for the selection and recruitment of nurses and midwives should be kept under review and should reflect current best practice. (7.65)

The Commission recommends that vacant permanent posts should be filled without delay. A framework should be put in place, following discussions between the Health Service Employers Agency and nursing unions, to ensure the problem (the number of long-term temporary nurses in the health services) does not recur. (7.66)

The Commission recommends that decisions on compassionate leave be delegated to local management so that there could be greater flexibility in granting additional compassionate leave, in appropriate cases. (7.67)

The Commission recommends the on-going development of occupational health programmes where they are currently provided and their introduction in areas of the health service where they are not currently available. (7.70)

The Commission recommends that the nursing unions and other relevant organisations establish a scheme to support nurses and midwives similar to the Sick Doctors Scheme. (7.72)

The Commission recommends that where critical incident debriefing systems are not in place they should be developed as a matter of urgency. (7.73)

The Commission recommends that all health service providers should ensure the availability of a professional confidential counselling system for nurses and midwives in their employment. (7.74)

The Commission recommends that nursing and midwifery management should be enabled to use their discretion to a greater extent to allow for greater flexibility in the provision of sick leave in certain exceptional circumstances. (7.75)

The Commission recommends that details of the scheme (for payment of an allowance and medical expenses to nurses or midwives assaulted during the course of work) be circulated generally. (7.75)

The Commission recommends that health service providers ensure the provision of adequate rest and changing facilities for nurses and midwives. (7.76)

The Commission recommends that if a nurse or midwife has acquired skills and experience abroad which are of value to the service, then a nurse or midwife manager should have sufficient discretion within budget to allow her or him to determine the point of entry on the incremental pay scale according to local priorities and needs. (7.77)

The Commission recommends that there should be long-term financial commitment to developing communication, management information and support systems to allow for greater devolution of budgets and staff development programmes. These programmes need to be underpinned by the allocation of adequate resources and a commitment to on-going funding. (7.78)

Nursing in the Community

8.1 This chapter outlines concerns in relation to the organisation and delivery of nursing services in the community. The consultative process undertaken by the Commission had identified a number of concerns in relation to the integration of nursing services in the community. There were also concerns in relation to the current and future role of public health nurses and community psychiatric nurses. The Commission makes recommendations in relation to the better integration of nursing services in the community, the organisation of nursing services and the role of nurses in the community. Midwifery services in the community are dealt with in chapter ten of the report.

8.2 The interim report of the Commission on Nursing identified a range of concerns in relation to the future direction of nursing in the community. Community psychiatric nurses and public health nurses have been working in the community since the 1960's. However, increasingly in recent years, a number of other nursing groups have started to work in the community, these include general, palliative care, psychiatric (other than community psychiatric nurses) mental handicap, practice nurses and other nurses. There was concern in relation to the level of integration of the increasingly diverse range of nursing services available in the community. Public health nurses were concerned in relation to their future direction with the increasing number of nursing groups providing services in the community. It was argued there was a need to examine the role of the Public Health Nurse (PHN) and to retain and develop the particular "community" skills which they had developed over the years and to examine the need for "specialist" skills in the community nursing service.

8.3 The Commission received from the Department of Health and Children a copy of the working party report on public health nursing, entitled *Public Health Nursing: A Review* (1997), which it considered in its deliberations on the issues identified in the interim report.

8.4 The Commission also requested Patricia Leahy-Warren, to undertake a literature review with the following terms of reference:

to conduct a review of the literature on community nursing - service models, care delivery, management of, education for and financing with particular reference to literature from the United Kingdom, United States of America, Australia, Canada and Europe, especially Finland.

8.5 The Commission requested Jean Clarke, Co-ordinator Higher Diploma in Nursing Studies (Public Health Nursing), Department of Nursing Studies, National University of Ireland - Dublin, Catherine McTiernan, Assistant Chief Nursing Officer, Mental Health Services, Eastern Health Board and Netta Williams, Royal College of Surgeons in Ireland, Department of General Practice to submit discussion documents outlining their views on a framework for the future development of nursing in the community.

An Outline of the Current Range of Nursing Services in the Community

Public Health Nursing

8.6 The current Public Health Nurse (PHN) service is based on a Department of Health circular in 1966 on the "District Nursing Service". The circular outlined the objectives of a community-based nursing service which were summarised as follows:

Broadly, the aim should be to make public health nurses available to individuals and to families in each area throughout the country. More specifically, the object should be to provide such domiciliary nursing, particularly for the aged; and at least equally important to attend to the public health care of children, from infancy to the end of the school going period. The nurses should provide health education in the home, and assist local medical practitioners in the care of patients who need nursing care but who do not require treatment in an institution - whether for medical or social reasons. The aim should be to integrate the district nursing service with the general practitioner, hospital, in-patient and out-patient services, so that the nurse will be able to fulfil the important function of an essential member of the community health team and carry out her duties in association with the hospital staff and others in her district.

8.7 The concept outlined in the circular was of a public health nursing role encompassing a broad range of preventive and caring functions. However, the role of the PHN has evolved in the thirty years since the circular of 1966. PHNs carry out a diverse range of nursing services responding to the needs of individuals, families and the community. The range of community services provided by PHNs includes:

- support and advice to a parent or parents following the birth of a child, such a service may be provided from shortly after the birth of the child and, if required, continues until the child is of school going age;

- the delivery of school health services;

- providing personalised nursing care to patients who have been discharged to the home from hospital;

- providing a range of nursing services to the elderly and support for carers in the home; and

- providing nursing services and support in the home for persons with a disability.

Health promotion remains an integral part of the role of the PHN. An example of the development of the role of PHN in recent years, which was cited in *Public Health Nursing: A Review* (1997), was the "Primary Health Care for Travellers Project" piloted by Pavee Point and the Eastern Health Board. The four aims of the project are to establish a model of traveller participation in the promotion of health; to liaise and assist in creating dialogue between travellers and health service providers in the area; and to highlight gaps in health service delivery to travellers and work towards reducing inequalities that exist in established services. Two co-ordinators, one a PHN and one a community worker, were appointed and eight traveller women were trained as community health workers. Such developments offer new opportunities for PHNs in meeting the particular health care needs of marginalised groups in the community.

8.8 The number of PHNs employed on 31 May, 1996 was 1,222 *(Public Health Nursing: A Review)*. PHNs are required to have a higher diploma in public health nursing provided by National University of Ireland - Dublin or National University of Ireland - Cork. Those applying to enter these programmes must be registered general nurses and midwives and also have at least two years work experience.

8.9 Whilst there is some variation between health boards, registered general nurses (RGNs) are employed to support the public health nursing service. In this capacity, they may cover weekend duties, twilight shifts or work as part of the community care team. They are also employed for periods of PHN absence. These RGNs are employed within the public health nursing system in a temporary capacity.

Mental Handicap Nursing

8.10 A substantial proportion of the mental handicap services are delivered by voluntary agencies serving catchment areas. Traditionally funding for these voluntary agencies was provided directly by the Department of Health. However, in line with *Shaping a Healthier Future* (1994), the Department of Health and Children published *Enhancing the Partnership* (1997) which provides for a new framework for the funding of voluntary mental handicap agencies. In future all voluntary mental handicap agencies will be funded through the health board in which they are based.

8.11   The emphasis of care in the mental handicap services is helping each client attain her or his potential as outlined in the report *Needs and Abilities* (1991). Nurses in this discipline have a diversity of roles, on a continuum ranging from intensive physical nursing of persons with a severe degree of handicap, to supportive guidance in the management of children, adults and the elderly. Client centred nursing services are provided in many settings including developmental day units, respite care, special education development, vocational training, adult special care units, long-term training units, residential services, including community-based group homes and community support services. Mental handicap nurses wish to see an expansion of the range of community services they provide with greater emphasis on the delivery of specialist mental handicap nursing care in the family home.

Psychiatric Nursing

8.12   Psychiatric nursing services are provided across a range of settings from acute hospitals to high support hostels to the community. This section is intended merely to outline the organisation of psychiatric services in the community which is just one element of the service. Psychiatric services are organised around catchment areas which in turn are divided into sectors to encompass a population of approximately 25,000. Inter-disciplinary teams were established to provide a range of services within each sector. Within this context there is no division between the hospital and community service, rather the hospital, health centre, day hospital and high support hostels are seen as options of care for clients within the catchment area. Psychiatric nurses can be based in any of these facilities. They manage a case load and provide a wide range of nursing services including rehabilitation, social skills training, individual counselling, group work, psycho-education, family support, liaison work and mental health education.

The Grade of Community Psychiatric Nurse

8.13   Community psychiatric nursing emerged as a feature of the Irish health services in the 1960's. During this period the development of new drugs for the treatment of certain conditions allowed for the discharge to the community of patients from mental health institutions. However, a number of such patients had to be readmitted to the institutions following the re-emergence of psychotic symptoms. The most significant reason for the return of such symptoms was identified as non-compliance with the new medication, together with poor preparation of the families to accept the recovered patient back home from the institution. In response to these and other needs the establishment of a new grade of Community Psychiatric Nurse (CPN) was deemed necessary to enable the smooth transition of patients from institutions into the community.

Practice Nurses

8.14   Practice nurses are a fairly recent development in the Irish health services. They are nurses attached to general practitioner practices and deliver a broad range of nursing services such as immunisations, women's health issues, ante natal care, wound care, counselling and asthma care. Practice nurses do not visit clients in their home. The scheme was set up by the Department of Health in 1989 to support general practitioners in their practice and there are now approximately 500 nurses attached to general practitioner practices. A subsidy towards the cost of employing a practice nurse is available to general practitioners participating in the General Medical Service (GMS) scheme with a patient panel size of at least 100. The amount of subsidy increases in bands of 100 with the maximum subsidy of £14,742 applicable to a GMS patient panel size of 1,200. This subsidy applies to practice nurses employed on a full-time basis and employment contracts of shorter duration are subsidised on a pro rata basis.

8.15 Palliative care nurses provide nursing care to chronically ill patients. The care provided by these nurses includes alleviation of pain, symptom control and enhancing quality of life. Palliative care nurses providing such a service may be based in the community. In recent years, hospice home care teams have been set up to provide a call-out and advisory service to enable families to care for a terminally ill family member at home.

Other Nurses

8.16 In addition to the nurses outlined above and the independent domiciliary midwives (referred to in chapter ten), other nursing groups have also recently begun to provide services in the community. Some are health board employees and some are employed by voluntary organisations or in the private sector.

A Framework for Improved Integration of Nursing Services in the Community

8.17 The increasingly diverse range of nursing services being provided in the community has resulted in calls for improved communication and integration between the range of nursing services in the community. The need for improved integration and co-operation in the delivery of nursing services in the community was identified as an issue during the consultative process undertaken by the Commission. It has also been stated that there is a need to improve communication between acute care and community care services. In the absence of improved integration and communication between those providing nursing services in the community, there is a danger that the delivery of nursing care will become increasingly fragmented which is not in the best interests of health service clients or the efficient utilisation of resources.

8.18 ***The Commission recommends that the Nursing and Midwifery Planning and Development Unit in each health board (see chapter seven of the report) should develop strategies to improve communication and integration between nursing services in community care areas.*** The systems developed by the Nursing and Midwifery Planning and Development Unit should recognise the particular social, demographic and geographic characteristics of each area. The functions of the Nursing and Midwifery Planning and Development Unit with reference to the community would include:

- developing, monitoring and reviewing the co-ordination and development of multi-disciplinary nursing services within a community care area;

- identifying inter-nursing disciplinary and inter-agency training needs and promoting the development of an inter-nursing disciplinary and inter-agency training strategy; and

- reviewing significant issues in relation to inter-nursing disciplinary and inter-agency co-operation arising from the handling of selected cases.

8.19 This monitoring role should ensure that on-going liaison and co-operation between the different services in the community are kept under constant review and will assist in the coming years in the fundamental reappraisal of nursing services in the community as outlined at the end of this chapter.

Issues Arising from the Consultative Process in Relation to Public Health Nursing

8.20 The Commission received numerous submissions from individual PHNs and from groups of PHNs expressing concern in relation to their role in the delivery of community health services during the consultative process. A number of issues were identified during the consultative process as being of concern to PHNs. These included:

- an increasing workload and an increasingly complex range of social and health issues related to substance abuse and child care protection; and

- concerns in relation to role reduction following the increasing emergence in the community of "specialist" nurses such as palliative care nurses and the increasing employment of practice nurses by general practitioners to provide nursing services attached to their practice.

8.21 Many of the issues identified in the consultative process have arisen as a result of substantial changes in the organisation and delivery of services since the Department of Health issued the circular establishing the current public health nursing system in 1966. The circular predates the establishment of the eight regional health boards under the Health Act 1970. Community nursing and general practitioner services had been closely aligned under the old dispensary scheme. The introduction of the choice of general practitioner scheme allowed patients in the General Medical Services system to choose their own doctor within the scheme. This has resulted in greater consumer choice. However, general practitioners are patient-based and work mainly in their surgeries, whereas PHNs are area-based and work mainly in the family home. This has resulted in increasing difficulty in aligning public health nursing services with general practitioner services in an area. There have also been further recent changes in the management of community services with the creation of general manager posts with responsibility for community care areas. Technological, social and epidemiological changes have also impacted on the role of the PHN.

8.22 The requirement that nurses applying for public health nursing have a midwifery qualification was also raised as an issue during the consultative process. It was felt by some that such a qualification may no longer be required because of the changed service demands currently facing PHNs. It was also seen as discouraging male nurses from becoming PHNs because of the very few who would have a midwifery qualification. It was suggested that an education module on maternity/child care might be incorporated in the public health nurse higher diploma programme as an alternative.

The Future Direction of Public Health Nursing

8.23 In considering the future direction of public health nursing, the Commission examined other international models for the delivery of nursing services in the community. However, the literature review undertaken by Patricia Leahy-Warren suggested that international trends do not offer any clear models or trends in the organisation and delivery of nursing in the community.

8.24 It appears that the public health nursing system is still essentially based on the Department of Health Circular of 1966. This circular is still seen by many as the core strategy statement in relation to the role of public health nursing in the community. The organisation and delivery of health services have changed radically since 1966 and there is a need to provide a revised strategy statement for public health nursing which has evolved substantially in the intervening thirty years as have other nursing and health services in the community. **The Commission recommends that the Department of Health and Children issue a revised strategy statement on the role of public health nursing. The report** Public Health Nursing: A Review (1997) **should inform the deliberations on a revised strategy statement.**

8.25   As stated previously the core concept of the public health nursing system is that of a nurse providing a wide range of nursing services to a district or area. The advantage of such a service was suggested as being the coherence of the nursing service provided to a diverse range of patients and clients in the community. In such a system an individual nurse can provide a range of services to a patient or family. It was suggested that a number of nurses responding to specific needs in a narrowly focused manner (such as would occur by a proliferation of specialists) brings with it the danger of increased fragmentation of the nursing service. Such fragmentation would cause particular problems in the community where distance and isolation from a health centre may already cause difficulties for patients and clients.

8.26   The Commission considers that the PHN should remain at the core of nursing services being delivered in the community. The PHN should remain focused on a district or area meeting the curative and preventive nursing needs of the population within the area. The Commission envisages the PHN continuing to be responsible for people of all ages and of every condition. However, the PHN will also act as a co-ordinator in the delivery of a range of services in the community. This co-ordination might also involve home nursing services provided by registered general nurses (the role of the registered general nurse in the community is discussed at paragraph 8.37). Consideration should be given to allowing the direct referral of clients to "specialist" services such as speech therapy, where such direct referral does not presently take place. There is also a need for public health nurses to develop to a greater extent their health promotion role. In order to fulfil the functions envisaged by the Commission, PHNs need to have their professional autonomy supported by the public health nursing management system. PHNs should also receive greater support in their role through the provision of new technology and, where appropriate, clerical support.

8.27   *The Commission recommends the continuation of the present area-based model of public health nursing. However, the PHN should be allowed focus to a greater extent on a health promotion and disease prevention role in the community. The Commission recommends that PHNs should receive greater support in their role through the provision of new technology and, where appropriate, clerical support.*

8.28   There is a need for improved links between the public health nursing system and other services in the community. In particular, there is a need for improved liaison and communication between public health nursing and general practitioners. A number of organisational factors appear to impact on good liaison between the two services. General practitioners are not health board employees and are patient based, whilst PHNs are health board employees and are area-based. These factors may make communication more difficult in urban areas in particular, where patients may have a greater choice of general practitioner. However, these organisational differences are not of themselves barriers to good communication and liaison. On a practical level health boards should give regular formal notification of the names of public health nurses to general practitioners in an area. PHNs should develop informal contacts and liaison with local general practitioners and practice nurses. The greater use of information technology would greatly assist communication, making it easier for both PHNs and general practitioners to contact each other. Good communication will require an active effort by both services to ensure the delivery of an optimal health service to their mutual patients.

8.29   Chapter six of the report has outlined a clinical career pathway in nursing involving clinical nurse specialists and advanced practitioners. The Commission considers that PHNs already operate at the level of clinical nurse specialist. The Commission considers that there is scope for the development of advanced practitioner roles in public health nursing.

8.30   As outlined previously the issue of the mandatory requirement of a midwifery qualification for entry to public health nursing was raised in the consultative process. The Board, in the publication *The Future of Nurse Education and Training in Ireland* (1994), having reviewed the evolving community care needs, recommended that the requirement of registration as a midwife should not be a prerequisite for entry to public health nursing. It recommended that it be replaced by a maternity and child care module. *Public Health Nursing: A Review* (1997) also recommended that the mandatory requirement of midwifery be discontinued (a minority of the Review Committee dissented). ***The Commission supports these views and recommends that, in light of the range of services offered by public health nurses and the on-going development of nursing and midwifery services in the community, registration as a midwife should no longer be a mandatory requirement for entry to the higher diploma in public health nursing or registration as a public health nurse. An alternative education programme relating more closely to the core generic maternal and child care service requirements of public health nursing should replace the mandatory midwifery requirement. The Commission recommends that the Board establish a working party composed of PHNs, health service providers and nurse educators to determine the content and duration of a course in maternal and child health as an alternative to the mandatory midwifery qualification.***

The Public Health Nursing Management Structure

8.31 There is a two tier management structure for public health nursing. The two management grades in public health nursing are Superintendent Public Health Nurse and Senior Public Health Nurse.

Superintendent Public Health Nurses

8.32 It was suggested during the consultative process that superintendent public health nurses, in common with other areas of nursing management, were excessively concerned with the detailed management of individual nurses rather than managing the function of nursing. This management of individual nurses may reflect the job description for superintendent public health nurses issued by the Department of Health and Children which describes their responsibilities as including the direction, supervision and co-ordination of public health nurses and other such staff as may be designated by the Chief Executive Officer. The Commission considers that superintendent public health nurses, in line with proposals in relation to senior nursing management, as outlined in chapter seven, need to provide strong professional leadership. There is a need for an increased focus on the strategic planning, quality assurance and professional development roles of the superintendent public health nurse. ***The Commission recommends that the future role of the superintendent public health nurse should be concentrated on issues such as:***

- ***providing strategic and clinical leadership and direction for nursing and related services which results in the delivery of effective, efficient, quality assured and patient centred nursing care;***

- ***developing a shared sense of commitment and participation amongst staff in the management of change, the development of nursing services and in responding to the changing health needs of patients;***

- ***developing the concept of care planning in collaboration with other professionals;***

- ***participating in the overall financial planning of the health service provided including the assessment of priorities in pay and non-pay expenditure;***

- ***ensuring that appropriate in-service education programmes and on-going learning needs are met for all assigned staff; and***

- ***ensuring that modern standards of clinical nursing care are in operation and that regular monitoring of nursing care is undertaken through audit.***

8.33   The Commission considers that in the modern health service environment the title Superintendent Public Health Nurse is slightly anachronistic. ***Therefore, the Commission recommends that the title of Superintendent Public Health Nurse be changed to Director of Public Health Nursing and that the job description reflect the changing role.***

Senior Public Health Nurses

8.34   The grade of Senior Public Health Nurse was introduced following a recommendation in the report of the *Working Party on General Nursing* in 1980. The working party envisaged that the senior public health nurse would be responsible for:

(i)   the implementation of policy by the routine organisation and management of the nursing services within that part of the community area allocated to her; and

(ii)   the co-ordination of the practical training programme of all students in that area.

However, it appears that the actual role of senior public health nurses may vary from area to area. A number of seniors specialise in areas such as child care or services for the elderly whilst others occupy a supporting management function within the public health nursing structure. There was much criticism of the management role of the senior public health nurse. It was suggested that many senior public health nurses performed no "real" management function and acted merely as conduits of information from public health nurses to superintendent public health nurses. There was even a suggestion given the type of administrative, "gatekeeping", non-decision making role assigned to many senior public health nurses that there was no longer any need to maintain the grade.

8.35   The Commission, in light of the re-focusing of the role of superintendent public health nurses, considers that there is an important management function to be fulfilled by senior public health nurses. In line with the original recommendation of the report of the *Working Party on General Nursing* (1980) and the report *Public Health Nursing: A Review* (1997), the routine management function of public health nursing should be assigned to senior public health nurses. There should be clear delegation of management responsibility and decision making in relation to specific geographic areas or specified functional roles to senior public health nurses. ***The Commission recommends that senior public health nurses should:***

- ***have a defined management role and not merely retain a "gatekeeping" administrative function;***

- ***have defined management responsibility with explicit delegation of authority;***

- ***have definite functional roles in managing areas for the delivery of public health nursing services; and***

- ***have the authority to manage their area of responsibility without constant reference to more senior management but, as in all management, there should be effective communication with public health nurses and senior management.***

8.36   The Commission considers that in the modern health service environment that the title Senior Public Health Nurse is slightly anachronistic. ***Therefore, the Commission recommends that the title of Senior Public Health Nurse be changed to Assistant Director of Public Health Nursing.***

Registered General Nurses working in the Community

8.37   The consultative process undertaken by the Commission had identified concerns amongst registered general nurses employed in the community at the lack of opportunities for permanent employment. Registered general nurses are currently employed in a temporary capacity when delivering nursing services in the community. The permanent employment of registered general nurses in the community nursing service has been recommended by a number of studies, including *The Working Party on General Nursing* (1980) and *Public Health Nursing: A Review* (1997). The principle is also supported in *The Interim Report of the Dublin Hospital Initiative Group* (1990) and *The Future of Nurse Education and Training in Ireland* (1994). *Public Health Nursing: A Review* states that *"the introduction of the general nurse will serve to improve the responsiveness of the service to patient/ client need."*

8.38 **The Commission recommends that where registered general nurses are employed in the community it should be in a permanent capacity in line with service need. Such nurses should be employed in support of the public health nursing service as part of the community nursing team. Flexible permanent part-time employment opportunities could be provided to registered general nurses working in the community which would more effectively align service needs with the personal circumstances of such nurses.** The focus of the registered general nurse could be on home nursing services provided in accordance with a care plan developed with the PHN. Prior to commencing work in the community, registered general nurses should be provided with in-service orientation training in community nursing.

Mental Handicap Nursing Services in the Community

8.39 As outlined previously, mental handicap nursing services are delivered primarily by voluntary agencies to a catchment area. There is a continuum of care from residential centres to high support hostels to day centres to support in the home of a client. The Commission envisages mental handicap services in the home of a client continuing to be provided under the aegis of a mental handicap service provider. Services radiate out from a residential centre and meet the entire range of mental handicap service needs, from institutional care to support in the home, as appropriate.

8.40 However, it appears from the consultative process that there is a need to further develop mental handicap nursing services to support clients in their home. The organisation and management of an enhanced community mental handicap nursing service should be encompassed within the existing management structures for the mental handicap services. There is a need to enhance the community service; the development of the clinical nurse specialist role within mental handicap will offer opportunities for the enhancement of community mental handicap services. Working titles for clinical nurse specialist in mental handicap nursing can be agreed between the National Council and health service providers when the posts are created.

8.41 There is a need to develop educational programmes to underpin the role of clinical nurse specialists in mental handicap services. Mental handicap will have a distinct identity within third-level institutes following the transition to the degree programme. Third-level institutes working in close collaboration with health service providers and the National Council should develop courses to underpin the enhancement of mental handicap services in the community.

8.42 The Commission also sees the potential for the development of advanced nurse practitioners in mental handicap nursing which will greatly enhance the delivery of services in the community and in residential care. These advanced practitioners would be educated to masters degree level, would practice an expanded nursing role, making professionally autonomous decisions and taking sole responsibility within agreed protocols.

8.43   *The Commission recommends that health service providers and the National Council examine the development of clinical specialisms with consequential posts which would enhance the delivery of mental handicap nursing services in the community.*

Psychiatric Nursing Services in the Community

8.44   As stated previously, psychiatric services are organised on a catchment area basis which are divided into sectors providing mental health services to population groups of 25,000. This allows the provision of a seamless service to the patient or client from the community to the hospital. A chief nursing officer is responsible for the management of psychiatric nursing services within the catchment area. In many sectors an assistant chief nursing officer is assigned to manage nursing services in the community.

8.45   The publication of *Planning for the Future* (1984) resulted in a reorientation of mental health services in this country with an even greater emphasis on community services. It was stated that increased numbers of psychiatric nurses were now working in the community and many CPNs in submissions to the Commission requested the continuance and review of the grade and their role.

8.46   The Commission supports the concept of a seamless psychiatric service covering acute centres, day hospitals, high support hostels and community services. The Commission envisages all psychiatric nurses being enabled to provide mental health services across the range of locations, including the community.

8.47   However, the Commission also recognises that there is a need for specialist community psychiatric nursing to further enhance the psychiatric nursing service provided in the community. There is an increasing need for an enhanced role for psychiatric nursing teams in the promotion of mental health and in areas such as suicide prevention. The psychiatric nursing service needs to extend its area of activity beyond responding to the needs of diagnosed patients and clients and towards enhancing the mental health of a population group within a geographic area. Community psychiatric nurse specialists should, in addition to holding a client group, focus on mental health promotion in the community. There is also a need to ensure the delivery of a high quality specialist nursing service to patients in the community who may have serious underlying mental illness. Such a service might include, for example, visiting schools in an area and providing advice and assistance to potentially vulnerable groups.

8.48   The Commission recommends the development of community psychiatric clinical nurse specialists. Such community psychiatric clinical nurse specialists have the same characteristics as clinical nurse specialists as outlined in chapter six. A specific grade for community psychiatric clinical nurse specialists should be developed and they should be designated "community mental health nurses".

8.49   The Commission envisages such community mental health nurses operating in a community psychiatric nurse team with registered psychiatric nurses. Such a team would meet the mental health needs of a community in a manner similar to a general nursing community care team composed of public health nurses and registered general nurses. The Commission considers the community mental health nurses as developing the role of the CPN and psychiatric nursing services in the community. CPNs who do not wish to convert to community mental health nurses would remain in their current position and on the same salary scale. However, for those CPNs who wish to seek an appointment as community mental health nurses, the Commission recommends that the interim procedures for the appointment of clinical nurse specialists, outlined in chapter six, would also apply to community mental health nurses.

8.50   The increasing prevalence and diversity of mental health needs in the community will also require the development of a role of advanced nurse practitioner in community psychiatric services. Advanced practitioners would be prepared to masters degree level and would see patients with undifferentiated and undiagnosed problems and initiate treatment within agreed parameters according to agreed protocols. This area should be examined by the National Council at an early stage. The Commission envisages that the development of such a service will greatly enhance the capacity of the psychiatric nursing services to respond flexibly and promptly to the growing mental health needs in the community. Career opportunities for psychiatric nurses in the community psychiatric services will also be available in management as outlined in chapter seven.

8.51   Educational programmes to underpin the role of the community mental health nurses and advanced nurse practitioner should be developed in a collaborative process involving third-level institutes, health service providers and the National Council as outlined in chapter six.

8.52   ***The Commission recommends that an enhanced community psychiatric nursing service should provide for the development of clinical nurse specialists and advanced practitioners within the community in each catchment area throughout the country, according to service need.***

Professional Support for Practice Nurses

8.53   Practice nurses in submissions to the Commission have requested a closer relationship with health boards to provide support for their professional development. The private contractual relationship between independent general practitioners and practice nurses is a unique relationship in nursing which offers numerous advantages to nursing. In addition to the support and assistance offered by general practitioners, the Commission considers that there is a need for improved support and assistance for practice nurses from health boards. ***The Commission recommends that the Nursing and Midwifery Planning and Development Unit in planning the continuing professional development needs of nurses within a health board area should also assist practice nurses in their professional development. The Commission also recommends that a practice nurse be attached on a sessional basis to the General Practice Unit within the health board to assist in identifying and supporting the development needs of practice nurses.*** The Commission recognises that the Irish College of General Practitioners has assisted practice nurses in their professional development and hopes that it will continue in this role.

The Future Direction of Nursing in the Community

8.54   The recommendations of the Commission, in relation to a future framework for public health nursing, mental handicap nursing, practice nursing and psychiatric nursing in the community, reflect the realities of the current state of development of nursing in the community in Ireland. However, the Commission considers that there is a need for a fundamental reappraisal of nursing services in the community as these services develop in the coming years. The demographic, social and health care changes which have impacted on nursing services in the community in the past thirty years will continue to alter the delivery and nature of nursing services in the community. The pace of change in the health services will mean that increasing numbers of patients and clients will need and seek nursing care in the community.

8.55   The Commission is conscious that the organisation and delivery of health services in the community is a complex and difficult task. The community presents a range of disparate needs which may vary substantially according to the demographic and socio-economic characteristics of a particular area. The community represents the environment in which nursing services are delivered but the service demands, priorities and difficulties will vary according to the particular local characteristics of the population.

8.56   The Commission is of the view that in the longer-term, consideration should be given to the development of a more coherent and integrated structure for the delivery of nursing services in the community. In particular, consideration should be given to the development of a more integrated management structure for nursing in the community. This more integrated management structure should encompass the range of nursing services provided in the community and allow for the creation of a post of "Director of Community Nursing". The holder of such a post would be responsible for the strategic planning and delivery of all nursing services in the community.

8.57   In addition to a more integrated management structure, a community nursing education programme could develop the community skills of each nursing discipline. Such a programme could provide a common core module on care and nursing within the framework of the broad band specialist community category, outlined in chapter six. Nurses might then progress by specialising in the care of particular client groups in the community. A common core community nursing programme would provide a common underpinning to all disciplines of nursing, practising in the community. Such a programme would provide nurses from each discipline with the necessary skills to function effectively in the community whilst being part of an inter-disciplinary community care team.

8.58   The outline framework for the greater integration of the management of and education for nursing in the community will require discussion in the profession. There is little consensus in the profession and amongst health service providers on the future direction of nursing in the community. There is a need for the profession to develop a coherent vision for the future direction of nursing in the community which reflects the nursing needs of the community rather than the status of individual groups within the profession.

Summary of Recommendations in Chapter Eight

The Commission recommends that the Nursing and Midwifery Planning and Development Unit in each health board (see chapter seven of the report) should develop strategies to improve communication and integration between nursing services in community care areas. (8.18)

The Commission recommends that the Department of Health and Children issue a revised strategy statement on the role of public health nursing. The report *Public Health Nursing: A Review* (1997) should inform the deliberations on a revised strategy statement. (8.24)

The Commission recommends the continuation of the present area based model of public health nursing. However, the public health nurse (PHN) should be allowed focus to a greater extent on a health promotion and disease prevention role in the community. The Commission recommends that PHNs should receive greater support in their role through the provision of new technology and where appropriate, clerical support. (8.27)

The Commission recommends that, in light of the range of services offered by PHNs and the on-going development of nursing and midwifery in the community, registration as a midwife should no longer be a mandatory requirement for entry to the higher diploma in public health nursing or registration as a public health nurse. An alternative education programme relating more closely to the core generic maternal and child care service requirements of public health nursing should replace the mandatory midwifery requirement. The Commission recommends that the Board establish a working party composed of PHNs, health service providers and nurse educators to determine the content and duration of a course in maternal and child health as an alternative to the mandatory midwifery qualification. (8.30)

The Commission recommends that the future role of the superintendent public health nurse should be concentrated on issues such as:

- providing strategic and clinical leadership and direction for nursing and related services which results in the delivery of effective, efficient, quality assured and patient centred nursing care;

- developing a shared sense of commitment and participation amongst staff in the management of change, the development of nursing services and in responding to the changing health needs of patients;

- developing the concept of care planning in collaboration with other professionals;

- participating in the overall financial planning of the health service provided including the assessment of priorities in pay and non-pay expenditure;

- ensuring that appropriate in-service education programmes and on-going learning needs are met for all assigned staff; and

- ensuring that modern standards of clinical nursing care are in operation and that regular monitoring of nursing care is undertaken through audit. (8.32)

The Commission recommends that the title of Superintendent Public Health Nurse be changed to Director of Public Health Nursing and that the job description reflect the changing role. (8.33)

The Commission recommends that senior public health nurses should:

- have a defined management role and not merely retain a "gatekeeping" administrative function;

- have defined management responsibility with explicit delegation of authority;

- have definite functional roles in managing areas for the delivery of public health nursing services; and

- have the authority to manage their area of responsibility without constant reference to more senior management, but as in all management, there should be effective communication with public health nurses and senior management. (8.35)

The Commission recommends that the title of Senior Public Health Nurse be changed to Assistant Director of Public Health Nursing. (8.36)

The Commission recommends that where registered general nurses are employed in the community it should be in a permanent capacity in line with service need. Such nurses should be employed in support of the public health nursing service as part of the community nursing team. Flexible permanent part-time employment opportunities could be provided to registered general nurses working in the community which would more effectively align service needs with the personal circumstances of such nurses. (8.38)

The Commission recommends that health service providers and the National Council examine the development of clinical nurse specialisms which would enhance the delivery of mental handicap nursing services in the community. (8.43)

The Commission recommends that an enhanced community psychiatric nursing service should provide for the development of clinical nurse specialists and advanced practitioners within the community in each catchment area throughout the country, according to service need. (8.52)

The Commission recommends that the Nursing and Midwifery Planning and Development Unit in planning the continuing professional development needs of nurses within a health board area should also assist practice nurses in their professional development. (8.53)

The Commission recommends that a practice nurse be attached on a sessional basis to the General Practice Unit within the health board to assist in identifying and supporting the development needs of practice nurses. (8.53)

Nursing in Care
of the Elderly
Chapter

9

Nursing in Care of the Elderly

9.1 Care of the elderly is not a nursing discipline but crosses most disciplines in nursing and is becoming an increasingly important component of the nursing service. Concern was expressed at the regional seminars, organised by the Commission following the publication of the interim report, that there had not been a section in the report on care of the elderly. The changing demographics of the Irish population mean that Ireland has an increasingly ageing profile. It was suggested that there was a need to emphasise the importance of this area of nursing. There was a concern that nursing in care of the elderly was viewed in some quarters as a "Cinderella" service. There was also concern about conditions and staffing levels in some care of the elderly settings which were adversely impacting on the quality of nursing care.

9.2 The Commission considers that care of the elderly offers substantial opportunities for nurse led services. Health boards and voluntary health service providers should examine to a greater extent the opportunity of developing nurse led services in care of the elderly. There is a need to promote care of the elderly as a career in nursing in order to continue to attract high calibre nurses into the service.

9.3 Care of the elderly facilities are located throughout the country and the Commission was conscious that in developing a clinical career pathway these services should provide further clinical career opportunities for nurses. The recommendation of the Commission on a clinical career pathway in nursing, outlined in chapter six, will provide clinical career opportunities in care of the elderly and not just in the highly technical, high patient turnover areas of nursing.

9.4 **The Commission** is concerned at the anecdotal information supplied to it in relation to conditions and staffing levels in care of the elderly and **recommends that the Department of Health and Children examine, as a matter of urgency, conditions and staffing levels in care of the elderly services**. Apart from the effect on the standards of care, staffing levels impact on the ability of staff to attend educational courses. **The Commission recommends that the Department of Health and Children review services for the elderly in each health board at the earliest opportunity.**

9.5 The setting up of post-registration nurse education programmes in care of the elderly is a welcome development. These courses vary in their academic award up to masters in gerontological nursing. The advancement of post-registration education to this level is important in relation to the development of clinical career pathways of clinical nurse specialist and advanced nurse practitioner in care of the elderly. Unfortunately, both the number of courses and their participants are small when compared with the number and educational needs of nurses working in care of the elderly. **The Commission recommends that centres of nursing education, in conjunction with third-level institutes, develop nurse education programmes to meet the needs of nurses working in care of the elderly, which would facilitate greater integration among the disciplines of nursing.**

9.6 Private nursing home bed provision has increased significantly according to a survey by the Department of Health in 1995. Nursing homes are covered in the Health (Nursing Homes) Act 1990, which allows for tighter quality controls through compulsory registration of nursing homes. In view of the significant increase in private nursing homes, the Commission considers that nurses working in these care of the elderly settings should be encouraged and facilitated to update their skills and knowledge. **The Commission recommends that application for or renewal of registration of nursing homes should indicate the opportunities for educational update provided for nursing staff.**

9.7   Care of the elderly nursing services are both hospital and community-based and span several disciplines of nursing. This diversity of service is identified in the substantial review by the National Council on Ageing and Older People in 1997 of the implementation of recommendations made in the Years Ahead Report (1988). The Commission was informed of the development of one such recommendation relating to the setting up of a psychiatry of old age service. This specialist development has encouraged a tailor made service for older people with functional mental illness and dementia, provided by a team involving community psychiatric nurses and psychiatric nurses in an integrated service. This service is seen as a valuable resource to all those collaborating in the delivery of care of the elderly services.

9.8   The 1997 review of the Years Ahead Report acknowledges the unique role of the PHN, in conjunction with the general practitioner, in the provision of care of the elderly at home. This role entails that PHNs, in their visits to the elderly, place emphasis on anticipatory care of the elderly, health promotion and care planning in collaboration with other community care services. To enable them in the provision of this role, PHNs need other supports such as RGNs, care assistants, home helps and other support services. **The Commission recommends that PHNs should receive greater support in their role in care of the elderly, through the provision of support staff and other services, where appropriate.**

9.9   As already identified, care of the elderly spans several nursing disciplines, based in the community and hospital services. This diversity requires a concerted effort to integrate and co-ordinate a comprehensive service for the elderly. The Commission considers that the Nursing and Midwifery Planning and Development Unit at health board level, in addition to creating specific posts within the service, will facilitate a further means of integrating and co-ordinating the diverse service for care of the elderly.

Summary of Recommendations in Chapter Nine

The Commission recommends that the Department of Health and Children examine, as a matter of urgency, conditions and staffing levels in care of the elderly services. (9.4)

The Commission recommends that the Department of Health and Children review services for the elderly in each health board at the earliest opportunity. (9.4)

The Commission recommends that centres of nursing education, in conjunction with third-level institutes, develop nurse education programmes to meet the needs of nurses working in care of the elderly, which would facilitate greater integration among the disciplines of nursing. (9.5)

The Commission recommends that application for or renewal of registration of nursing homes should indicate the opportunities for educational update provided for nursing staff. (9.6)

The Commission recommends that PHNs should receive greater support in their role in care of the elderly, through the provision of support staff and other services, where appropriate. (9.8)

Certain Issues Relating to Mental Handicap Nursing, Midwifery and Sick Children's Nursing

Chapter

10

Certain Issues Relating to Mental Handicap Nursing, Midwifery and Sick Children's Nursing

10.1   This chapter considers particular issues relating to mental handicap nursing, midwifery and sick children's nursing. The substantive issues relating to the clinical disciplines of general and psychiatric nursing are addressed throughout the report. Recommendations made throughout the report are also relevant to mental handicap nursing, midwifery and sick children's nursing. However, there are a number of issues relating to mental handicap nursing, midwifery and sick children's nursing which are particular to each of the disciplines. Mental handicap and sick children's nursing are viewed by some as low profile disciplines that require particular promotion. Midwifery has an identity distinct from nursing and there are a number of issues in relation to the preparation for and practice of midwifery. Issues in relation to the regulation of midwifery have been addressed in chapter four. This chapter seeks to provide a framework in relation to the future direction of mental handicap nursing, midwifery and sick children's nursing.

Mental Handicap Nursing

10.2   Services for people with a mental handicap (also referred to as intellectual disability) have evolved in recent years with a greater emphasis on integration at school, work and in the community. The mental handicap nurse works with all age ranges and all levels of handicap including persons with mild, moderate, severe, profound and multiple handicaps. The age range includes an increasing population of senior citizens. A wide range of services, are provided, such as:

- day care including assessments, early intervention services, pre-school, special education development;

- residential and respite care, which is inclusive of community group houses and local centres; and

- vocational training, sheltered and supported employment.

10.3   A number of submissions suggested that the role of the mental handicap nurse needed to be clearly defined in an increasingly diverse and complex service for those with such a handicap. There was a need to respond to changes taking place within the service such as the increasing age profile and increasingly complex range of disabilities of those with a mental handicap. Submissions referred to the need for nurses to be at the centre of the service, responding to these changing needs and suggested that the skills of the mental handicap nurse needed to be retained and developed to ensure the on-going development of a quality and responsive service. Some mental handicap nurses expressed concern in relation to a lack of appreciation of their specialist skills with the increasing employment of general nurses, teachers and non-nursing personnel in these services.

10.4   The Commission received a copy of the *Report of the Working Group on the Role of the Mental Handicap Nurse* from the Department of Health and Children. The Commission also visited Stewarts Hospital, Palmerstown and St. Joseph's Hospital, Clonsilla to meet with mental handicap nurses.

10.5   The Commission, having reflected on the service needs in the mental handicap services, in particular as identified in the *Annual Report of the National Intellectual Disability Database Committee (1996)* considered that there was a need to stress the crucial importance of mental handicap nurses to the service. Nurses from this discipline provide a range of services across a wide variety of locations to meet the particular, complex and difficult needs of their clients. Meeting these needs requires a high level of intuitive and perceptual skills which can only be acquired through experience and a

10

dedicated education programme. The quality of the service provided to this most vulnerable group of clients, who will remain in need of support and care from infancy to late adulthood, is primarily determined by the quality of the nursing care. The Commission recognises that mental handicap nurses require particular skills and personal qualities distinct from those in other disciplines of nursing. The Commission has already recommended that mental handicap nursing remain a direct entry discipline with a four year third-level institute-based degree programme in chapter five. *The Commission considers that there is a need to promote the distinct identity and unique working environment of mental handicap nursing and recommends that the Board develop a strategy, in consultation with nurse educators, mental handicap nurses and service providers, to promote mental handicap nursing as a career.*

10.6   It was submitted to the Commission that nurses have been employed as houseparents in the mental handicap services and have carried out duties which could be characterised as nursing duties. They have later discovered that their service was not recognised as nursing service. The Commission considers that the question of their professional status should be reviewed by the parties concerned.

10.7   The issue of the increasing use of non-nursing personnel in the mental handicap services was also raised during the consultative process. There was a view that the increasing use of non-nursing personnel combined with a shortage of mental handicap nurses was contributing towards an increasing "de-professionalisation" of the service. The better promotion of mental handicap nursing combined with the move to a degree qualification on registration should assist in improving the profile and attractiveness of mental handicap nursing in the longer-term. However, the Commission also considers that there is a need for the Department of Health and Children to examine the policies and practices of mental handicap service providers in relation to non-nursing personnel.

Midwifery

10.8   It was argued by some midwives during the consultative process that the Nurses Act 1985, which governs the regulation of the nursing profession, fails to recognise the separate and unique role of midwives by defining a nurse as also including a midwife. It was argued that midwives had a distinct role in the delivery of care to women during the course of pregnancy and following birth. Many European countries offer direct entry into midwifery and midwifery students are not registered general nurses in those countries. Midwifery training and practice are dealt with under a separate EU Directive, 80/155/EEC.

10.9   The definition of a midwife adopted by the International Confederation of Midwives (ICM) and the International Federation of Gynaecologists and Obstetricians (FIGO), in 1972 and 1973 respectively and later adopted by the World Health Organisation (WHO) was given in a number of submissions to the Commission. The definition was amended by the ICM in 1990 and the amendment ratified by the FIGO and the WHO in 1991 and 1992 respectively and now reads:

"A midwife is a person who, having been regularly admitted to a midwifery educational programme, duly recognised in the country in which it is located, has successfully completed the prescribed course of studies in midwifery and has acquired the requisite qualifications to be registered and/or legally licensed to practice midwifery. She must be able to give the necessary supervision, care and advice to women during pregnancy, labour and postpartum period, to conduct deliveries on her own responsibility and to care for the newborn and the infant. This care includes preventative measures, the detection of abnormal conditions in mother and child, the procurement of medical assistance and the execution of emergency measures in the absence of medical help. She has an important task in health counselling and education, not only for the women, but also within the family and the community. The work should involve antenatal education and preparation for parenthood and extends to certain areas of gynaecology, family planning and child care. She may practise in hospitals, clinics, health units, domiciliary conditions or in any other service."

10.10　Many midwives during the consultative process expressed the view that midwifery practice had become increasingly constrained in recent years and that midwives were becoming de-skilled in the provision of maternity services. Many midwives suggested that the increasing "medicalisation" of normal pregnancies had turned midwives into obstetric nurses rather than the independent practitioners allowed by their education. It was suggested that midwifery provided substantial scope for the development of a woman centred care service before, during and after pregnancy. In order for midwifery to develop its potential for the delivery of women centred care, it was suggested that the regulatory framework for nursing practice needed to recognise the distinct identity of midwives. In addition, there were concerns in relation to the current education programme for the preparation of midwives. The current programme is of two years duration, with thirteen weeks theoretical instruction. Students are part of the midwifery workforce during the two year period. Concern was also expressed during the consultative process in relation to the provision and supervision of a domiciliary midwifery service.

10.11　The Commission recognises that midwifery has an identity distinct from nursing. Midwives respond to the needs of pregnant women, many of whom are increasingly aware of the birth options available to them. Midwifery offers practitioners a unique opportunity for autonomous practice in the provision of health services to women. The Commission has outlined in chapter four its recommendations in relation to a revised regulatory framework for midwifery and has recommended that future amending legislation recognise the distinct identity of midwives.

The Education of Midwives

10.12　The two year programme for the education of midwives commenced in 1983 and there are increasing concerns that it may no longer adequately prepare midwives to meet the service needs of the next century. In particular, there are concerns that midwives are being trained as "obstetric" nurses and do not have the preparation necessary to develop as autonomous practitioners. There is an increasing international demand for intervention free maternity services. The Commission, during a visit to Australia, visited a midwife led birth centre attached to a maternity hospital in the Central Sydney Area Health Services (there is no similar service attached to a maternity hospital in Ireland). If midwives were to offer similar intervention free maternity services in Ireland, it has been suggested that there would need to be an improved educational programme for entry to midwifery. It has been argued that the thirteen weeks of theoretical instruction provided to student midwives is inadequate. **The Commission recommends that the Board review the current midwifery education programme as a matter of urgency. The review should, in particular, examine the length of the programme and the level of theoretical instruction provided to student midwives and compare such theoretical instruction with that required under a third-level post graduate higher diploma programme. In addition, the Commission recommends that a direct entry midwifery course be piloted by the Board in a maternity hospital. Such a programme should initially be provided at diploma level but should move to a degree programme in 2002.**

Domiciliary Midwifery

10.13　A number of midwives have set up independent private practice around the country to provide a midwifery service for those wishing to have a homebirth. These midwives contract directly with the woman wishing to have a homebirth. The fee may range from £600 to £900. There are fourteen independent domiciliary midwives in Ireland.

10.14　Concern was expressed during the consultative process in relation to the current supervisory arrangements for domiciliary midwives providing for homebirths. Health boards are obliged, under the Health Act 1970, to provide domiciliary midwifery care for women who wish to give birth at home. It was reported that in 1996, there were 50,390 births in Ireland, of which 206 were home

10

births (CSO, 1996). Section 57(1) of the 1985 Act provides that if a midwife intends to practise in a health board area, she must notify the health board of her intention to practise if she is not an employee of the health board. Section 57(2) of the 1985 Act imposes a duty on health boards to exercise general supervision and control over independent midwives practising in a health board area. The person designated by health boards to exercise this supervision and control is a superintendent public health nurse. There was concern expressed by superintendent public health nurses and midwives in relation to this arrangement.

10.15   The Commission considers that the determination of the suitability of midwives to provide an independent domiciliary service and the professional parameters of their practice are matters for the Board. *The Commission recommends that the statutory midwives committee within the Board, proposed in the revised regulatory framework, develop a scope of practice framework covering the activities of independent midwives in the community. Such a scope of practice should cover the professional requirements of a midwife practising in the community and address issues in relation to their on-going practice and clinical audit. The Commission recommends the deletion of section 57(2) of the 1985 Act.*

Sick Children's Nursing

10.16   Sick children's nursing appears to have a particularly low profile as a separate discipline within the nursing profession. The Commission did not receive a large number of submissions from nurses practising in this area and had difficulty sourcing material in relation to the historical background to the discipline.

10.17   It was suggested by registered sick children's nurses during the consultative process, that nursing children differs from nursing adults because of children's special health care needs. It was submitted that children were physically and emotionally different from adults and needed constant care and support from their parents. Children, therefore, required care from specially skilled staff. Because of the age range of patients, sick children's nurses required an in-depth understanding of the physical, psychological, social development and maturation processes from infancy to early adulthood. Sick children's nurses needed acute skills of observation and communication as frequently their patients were not capable of telling them what was wrong with them and might be totally dependent on them. It was submitted that in promoting the concept of family centred care, the sick children's nurse required special skills in teaching and support by entering into partnership with families in the provision of care. There have been social changes in the nature of the family in Ireland in recent years which have challenged traditional concepts of family life and impacted on the nursing care provided to children. Some parents of children in hospital could themselves be considered children, being under eighteen years of age.

10.18   The care of children suffering from medical problems requires nurses who have the training and education to respond to their particular emotional and physical requirements. Sick children's nursing is at the core of the paediatric services. The Commission has recommended an increase in the number of sick children's nurses on the Board to start the process of raising the profile of the discipline. However, there is a need for directors of nursing from the paediatric hospitals, sick children's nurse educators and nurses in the paediatric services to develop a coherent vision for the future development of the discipline.

The Education of Sick Children's Nurses

10.19   The education of sick children's nurses recently became a post-registration education qualification. It is an eighteen month course open to nurses who are already on the register with the Board. Previously there had been direct entry courses in sick children's nursing and it seems that a key factor in the move to a post-registration qualification was the increasing difficulty in recruiting students. Many nurses, with only a sick children's nursing qualification, had found it difficult to get employment outside the major Dublin paediatric hospitals. Developments in medical diagnoses and therapeutics meant that acutely ill children, who might not previously have survived, were now being cared for by sick children's nurses. It was also suggested that the nature of sick children's nursing and the changing nature of the family, with an increasing number of single teenage parents, required a greater maturity in the practice of sick children's nursing. It was suggested that with the development of degree programmes for direct entry nursing disciplines there may be duplication between the current sick children's nursing programme and the pre-registration degree programmes. It was suggested that the sick children's nursing programme could be shortened to twelve months.

10.20   *The Commission recommends that the qualification of sick children's nursing remain a post-registration qualification. However, prior to the transition of direct entry nursing disciplines to a degree programme, directors of nursing from the paediatric hospitals, sick children's nurse educators and the Board should review the content, duration and academic award of the sick children's nursing course, in light of the proposed degree course curricula.*

10.21   It was suggested that the title Sick Children's Nurse was slightly anachronistic in the modern health service. *The Commission accepted this view and recommends that the title Sick Children's Nurse be changed to Child Health Nurse.*

10

Summary of Recommendations in Chapter Ten

The Commission considers that there is a need to promote the distinct identity and unique working environment of mental handicap nursing and recommends that the Board develop a strategy, in consultation with nurse educators, mental handicap nurses and service providers, to promote mental handicap nursing as a career. (10.5)

The Commission recommends that the Board review the current midwifery education programme as a matter of urgency. The review should, in particular, examine the length of the programme and the level of theoretical instruction provided to student midwives and compare such theoretical instruction with that required under a third-level post graduate higher diploma programme. In addition, the Commission recommends that a direct entry midwifery course be piloted by the Board in a maternity hospital. Such a programme should initially be provided at diploma level but should move to a degree programme in 2002. (10.12)

The Commission recommends that the statutory midwives committee within the Board, proposed in the revised regulatory framework, develop a scope of practice framework covering the activities of independent midwives in the community. Such a scope of practice should cover the professional requirements of a midwife practising in the community and address issues in relation to their on-going practice and clinical audit. (10.15)

The Commission recommends the deletion of section 57(2) of the 1985 Act, (which places a duty on health boards to exercise general supervision and control over independent midwives practising in a health board area). (10.15)

The Commission recommends that the qualification of sick children's nursing remain a post-registration qualification. However, prior to the transition of direct entry nursing disciplines to a degree programme, directors of nursing from the paediatric hospitals, sick children's nurse educators and the Board should review the content, duration and academic award of the sick children's nursing course, in light of the proposed degree course curricula. (10.20)

The Commission recommends that the title Sick Children's Nurse be changed to Child Health Nurse. (10.21)

Other Issues

Chapter

11

Other Issues

11.1　This chapter considers two further issues identified as being of concern to nurses and midwives during the consultative process. Firstly, the Commission outlines various aspects related to retirement problems which were communicated to the Commission on Public Service Pensions for consideration within the context of its terms of reference. Secondly, the Commission outlines a possible approach in relation to bullying. However, it is hoped that other proposed developments previously outlined in the report may also assist in resolving this issue, which should not be viewed in isolation.

Retirement

11.2　This section of the report deals with the retirement and pension issues which nurses and midwives asked the Commission on Nursing to address during the consultative process.

Issues Arising During the Consultative Process

11.3　Chapter Seven of the interim report of the Commission on Nursing identified many concerns which nurses and midwives held in relation to pensions and retirement; a summary of the main issues is given below:

- it was highlighted that as nursing and midwifery are a predominantly female profession, the years spent out of employment raising a family are lost to nurses in calculating pension entitlement;

- the effect of the marriage bar, on early retirement prospects, for those now in the forty-five to sixty-five age group, was brought to the attention of the Commission. It was reported, that on the removal of the marriage bar, many married nurses and midwives returned to the workforce, but with broken years of service for the purpose of calculating pension entitlement. In addition, if the nurse or midwife is to benefit from a reasonable pension at retirement, they may be faced with the requirement to repay a marriage gratuity plus compound interest on the sum accruing over the intervening period;

- nurses and midwives argued that there is inequity between the years of service required for pension purposes in the psychiatric service and the years required by other disciplines within the profession. Nurses and midwives sought parity with psychiatric nurses who are entitled to have each year of service after twenty years count as two years for pension purposes. This enables them to have thirty years service reckonable as forty years service for retirement purposes and to retire, if they so wish, with immediate payment of pension at fifty-five years of age;

- because of the physically arduous and stressful nature of the work, nurses and midwives submitted that there was a need for all nurses to have access to early retirement if required;

- many nurses and midwives felt aggrieved that years of service in the profession worked abroad, were not acknowledged for superannuation purposes in Ireland, making it very difficult for some nurses to have enough years to avail of early retirement schemes or to have a reasonable occupational pension on retirement;

- some nurses and midwives reported that if they had undertaken their training or worked when qualified in a private hospital, those years were not reckonable for public service superannuation purposes;

- it was submitted that calculating pensionable allowances on the basis of an average of the amounts received in the last three years of service can be unfair, as it places undue pressure on nurses and midwives to optimise premium payments in the final years of service;

- nurses and midwives described the financial effect of the conversion process from long-term temporary to permanent contracts. For nurses and midwives with considerable temporary service, it is compulsory to pay superannuation contributions for their years of temporary service, when taking permanent employment;

- a plea was made by nurses and midwives for more flexible employment arrangements. It was reported that many nurses and midwives who left employment to raise families or for other reasons would like the opportunity to return to nursing or midwifery in a permanent part-time capacity. It was suggested that a barrier to the introduction of permanent part-time employment opportunities was the difficulty in relation to pension entitlement for part-time public service workers;

- some nurses and midwives submitted that information about pension entitlements should be made available to nurses and midwives early in their career to allow sufficient time to make provision for future requirements; and

- requests were made for pre-retirement programmes to be more widely provided for by employers.

Retirement Initiatives

11.4 The claim in relation to early retirement for nurses (other than psychiatric nurses) and midwives was considered by an Adjudication Board during the negotiations on pay and conditions of nurses and midwives in early 1997, which was then considered by the Labour Court. The Board and the Labour Court recommended that all of the arguments be considered by the Commission on Public Service Pensions (CPSP) in the context of its terms of reference. However in the interim, the Labour Court recommended the implementation of a limited initiative from January 1997 to address the immediate situation of nurses and midwives (other than nurses and midwives who already enjoy enhanced superannuation terms), who find the demands of the profession are such that they are no longer able to function at the level of professional performance they themselves and management require (LCR15450). The Court recommended that:

- an early retirement facility be introduced for nurses and midwives, aged fifty five or over with at least thirty five years service, subject to a number of criteria which would underpin the delivery of a consistently high quality nursing service, limited to a quota of 200 per annum, to operate on a pilot basis pending the report of the CPSP; and

- the introduction of a pre-retirement initiative to facilitate nurses and midwives in reducing the amount of actual service commitment in the years immediately preceding their retirement. Nurses and midwives, aged fifty five or over, who have twenty years whole-time service and who do not otherwise enjoy enhanced superannuation benefits, may make application to work on a job-sharing basis for a maximum of three years prior to retirement, with the three years in question, or other lesser period, to reckon as full-time service for superannuation purposes. A quota not exceeding 600 applications was set for the initial three years operation of the scheme with up to a maximum of 300 applications being approved in year one.

11.5 It appears that there is generally a low uptake of the scheme. By early 1998 approximately eleven applications were made for early retirement and sixteen applications for the pre-retirement scheme.

Commission on Public Service Pensions

11.6 The Commission on Public Service Pensions was established in February 1996 with the following terms of reference:

"to examine and report on the pension terms of public servants employed in the Civil Service (non-industrial and industrial), Defence Forces, Gardaí, Education, Health and Local Authority Services, having regard to:

(1) the present and future costs arising under the schemes financed by the Exchequer;

(2) claims for improvements in existing scheme benefits, including claims for voluntary early retirement;

(3) changes in the working environment and conditions of employment of public servants since the schemes were introduced; and

(4) the operational needs of the Services concerned."

The Commission on Public Service Pensions submitted an interim report to the Minister for Finance in August 1997.

11.7 The Commission considers that The Public Services Pension Commission (CPSP) in its examination of the totality of pension issues within the public service is in a better position to examine the difficult and complex pensions/retirement issues identified as being of concern to nurses and midwives during the consultative process. For this reason the **Commission wrote to the CPSP outlining in detail the concerns of nurses and midwives in relation to retirement issues. The Commission understands that the CPSP is considering these issues within the context of its terms of reference.**

Options to Increase Pension Entitlement

11.8 The Commission was concerned that, during the consultative process, many nurses and midwives appeared unaware of the options available to them to increase their pension entitlement. These options may be availed of at the individual initiative of a nurse or midwife. Nurses and midwives need to take individual responsibility for planning their retirement. It is important for every nurse and midwife to understand what their pension/retirement entitlements will be, based on their work pattern and the level of pensionable service which they can expect to have, at retirement age. The options available to nurses and midwives to increase their pension entitlement include the purchase of notional service (to a maximum of forty years) or the purchase of additional voluntary contributions (AVCs). The option most suited to an individual will depend on her or his circumstances. However, details in relation to the purchase of notional years or additional voluntary contributions should be available from either the personnel section within a health service provider or a nursing trade union. **The Commission considers that health service providers have a responsibility in assisting nurses and midwives to plan their retirement by prompting discussion and making available information on the retirement and pension options which are readily available.**

Bullying

11.9 Many nurses and midwives in discussions at the consultative fora and in written submissions complained of bullying in the workplace. A definition of bullying provided to the Commission by the Manufacturing Science Finance union was that it involved *"persistent, offensive, abusive, intimidating, malicious or insulting behaviour, abuse of power or unfair penal sanctions, which makes the* *recipient feel upset, threatened, humiliated or vulnerable, which undermines their self-confidence and which may cause them to suffer stress."* Bullying can have an adverse impact on the victim who may suffer chronic anxiety and stress which may result in the loss of self-confidence, ill-health and mental distress. It is not necessarily characterised by overt aggression or violence but in many cases may take the form of a continuous series of covert and manipulative actions which have the effect of undermining the self-confidence and personality of the victim. The Irish Business and Employers Confederation gave examples of bullying behaviour as including:

- abusing a position of power by unnecessarily undermining the work of a colleague and/or placing unreasonable demands on a particular individual;

- unreasonable or inappropriate monitoring of the performance of a colleague;

- persistently setting objectives with unreasonable or impossible deadlines or unachievable tasks;

- persistent negative attacks on personal or professional performance without good reason or legitimate authority;

- spreading malicious rumours or allegations;

- continually overriding the authority of a person;

- freezing out, ignoring or excluding; and

- shouting, aggressive behaviour, impatience, insults, etc.

11.10   It appeared from the views expressed by nurses during the consultative process that bullying may be taking place at a variety of levels in nursing and midwifery. The Commission heard of complaints of bullying from students, staff nurses and midwives and from management.

11.11   Bullying is not a phenomenon peculiar to nursing and midwifery. It is a form of harassment in the workplace that has been a source of concern to both employers and unions. The Commission understands that discussions are taking place between the Health Service Employers Agency, health boards and the nursing unions to formulate an agreed approach to bullying. Similarly, the Commission understands that the Irish Business and Employers Confederation is in the process of drafting guidelines for members to combat bullying in the workplace. **The Commission recommends that all health service employers develop formal and informal procedures to deal with bullying in the workplace.** Informal procedures may be sufficient to resolve a complaint at local level with a minimum of disturbance. Where these are not effective, formal procedures should be implemented. All managers and nurses should be made fully aware of the procedures.

Summary of Recommendations in Chapter Eleven

The Commission recommends that all health service employers develop formal and informal procedures to deal with bullying in the workplace. (11.11).

*Implementation of
the Recommendations
of the Commission on Nursing*

Chapter

12

Implementation of the Recommendations
of the Commission on Nursing

12.1   The Commission has made a wide range of recommendations which are of major importance to the future development of nursing and midwifery. There is a need to ensure that the profession is involved in the implementation of the recommendations of the Commission. There should be clear communication with the profession on the implementation of the recommendations which will have a fundamental impact on the daily working lives of nurses and midwives.

12.2   *Therefore, the Commission recommends the establishment of a monitoring committee under the aegis of the Department of Health and Children comprising representatives of the Department, the Board, the four nursing unions and service providers to monitor the progress of the implementation of the recommendations. The Commission recommends that progress reports on the implementation of the recommendations be prepared annually for circulation among the profession.*

12.3   The Commission recognises that the recommendations contained in the report need to be implemented in a structured, phased and carefully planned manner. This needs to be balanced against the need of the profession to see progress at an early stage in response to the report of the Commission. The Commission is of the view that this balance can best be achieved by setting a target date for the implementation of all the recommendations in the report and by suggesting a timetable for certain key institutional and structural reforms. *The Commission is of the view that all the recommendations contained in the report should be implemented by the end of 2002 at the latest.* Some of the recommendations contain a time scale for their implementation. Those that do not have a time scale should be implemented as soon as is practicable. *The Commission recommends the following timetable in relation to certain key institutional and structural reforms:*

Regulation of the Profession

- The legislation amending the Nurses Act 1985 should be introduced before the Houses of the Oireachtas by early 1999.

- The working party, composed of the Department of Health and Children, the Health Service Employers Agency, nursing and other appropriate organisations, to establish criteria in relation to entry requirements, education qualifications and training for care assistants, should be established by January, 1999.

Preparation for the Profession

- The forum composed of representatives of the third-level institutes, schools of nursing, health service providers and the Board should be established at the earliest possible date. It is to report within two years of its establishment and a lead in time is required following its report to allow nurse educators, career guidance counsellors and others prepare for the transition to the pre-registration degree programme at the start of the academic year in 2002.

- The Board should begin discussions with the CAO to allow the nursing application process to be incorporated within the CAO system in time for the intake of students in the year 2000.

- The degree programme should commence at the start of the academic year in 2002. As stated in the report, no third-level institute should commence a pre-registration degree programme in advance of this date. All third-level institutes and each of the direct entry disciplines (general, mental handicap and psychiatric nursing) should start the degree programme in 2002.

Professional Development

- The National Council for the Professional Development of Nursing and Midwifery is a core recommendation of the Commission. It is important that the National Council be established at the earliest possible date. The clinical career pathway for nurses and midwives proposed by the Commission is dependent on the effective operation of the National Council. It is important that the National Council commences its work in determining areas of specialism in nursing and midwifery and the guidelines for the creation of specialist posts.

- The Commission is aware that a number of the profession are already operating at the level of specialist. Some of these have developed in an ad-hoc manner as outlined in the report. It is important that the position of specialist posts be regularised at an early date. Top priority should be given to the creation of clinical nurse or midwife specialist and advanced nurse or midwife practitioner posts. The Commission envisages that the initial such posts will have been created by the end of 1999 at the latest.

Role of Nurses and Midwives in the Management of Services

- The Chief Nursing Officer at the Department of Health and Children will have a crucial role in the implementation of the recommendations of the Commission. The appointment of additional support staff recruited by the Department of Health and Children to assist in the implementation of the report should be one of the first initiatives undertaken in response to the report.

- Another key recommendation is the establishment of a Nursing and Midwifery Planning and Development Unit in each health board. The units will have a range of functions and are seen as providing a crucial strategy development and planning function at a time of substantial change within the profession. In particular they have an important role to play in the creation of clinical nurse or midwife specialist and advanced nurse or midwife practitioner posts. Therefore it is important that these units are put in place at the earliest possible date.

References,
Bibliography, Appendices
and Acknowledgements

References

Advisory Committee on Training in Nursing (1995) *Recommendations on Continuing and Specialist Education and Training* III/F5004/5/93-EN. Brussels: Commission of the European Communities.

Alberta Association of Registered Nurses (1989) Position Paper on Graduate Education in Nursing. AARN April, 25-26.

An Bord Altranais (1997) *Continuing Professional Education for Nurses in Ireland: A Framework.* Dublin: An Bord Altranais.

An Bord Altranais (1997) *Guidance to Nurses and Midwives on the Administration of Medical Preparations.* 4th Ed. Dublin: An Bord Altranais.

An Bord Altranais (1997) Report for the Year 1996: *Auditors Report and Financial Statements for 1996.* Dublin: An Bord Altranais.

An Bord Altranais (1994) *The Future of Nurse Education and Training in Ireland.* Dublin: An Bord Altranais.

An Bord Altranais (1991) *Nurse Education and Training: Consultative Document.* Interim report of Bord Altranais. Dublin: An Bord Altranais.

An Bord Altranais (1988) Nurses Rules (as amended) in An Bord Altranais (1994) *Rules for the Education and Training of Student Nurses.* Dublin: An Bord Altranais.

An Bord Altranais (1988) *The Code of Professional Conduct for Each Nurse and Midwife.* Dublin: An Bord Altranais.

Audit Commission (1992) *Making Time for Patients: A Handbook for Ward Sisters.* London: HMSO.

Benner, P., Tanner, C. and Chesla, C. (1996) *Expertise in Nursing Practice-caring, clinical judgement and ethics.* New York: Springer Publishing Company.

Benner, P. (1984) From Novice to Expert: *Excellence and Power in Clinical Nursing.* Menlo Park: Addison-Wesley.

Cameron Buccheri, R. and Ogier, M.E. (1994) The USA's Nurse Managers and UK's Ward Sister: Critical Roles for Empowerment. *Journal of Clinical Nursing* 3, 205-211.

Castledine, G. (1995) Defining Specialist Nursing. *British Journal of Nursing* 4(5), 264-265.

Central Statistics Office (1998) *Quarterly National Household Survey.* Dublin: Stationary Office.

Central Statistics Office, Provisional figures for home births (1996) (Unpublished).

Clarke, J., Warr, J. (1995) Improved by Degrees. *Nursing Times* 91(37), 51-53.

Council of European Communities (1989) Council Directive (89/595/EEC) amending Directive 77/452/EEC concerning the mutual recognition of diplomas, certificates and other evidence of the formal qualifications of nurses responsible for general care, including measures to facilitate the effective exercise of the right of establishment and freedom to provide services, and amending Directive 77/453/EEC concerning the co-ordination of provisions laid down by law, regulation or administrative action in respect of the activities of nurses responsible for general care.

Council of European Communities (1980) Council Directive (80/155/EEC) concerning the mutual recognition of diplomas, certificates and other evidence of qualification in midwifery and including measures to facilitate the effective exercise of the right of establishment and freedom to provide services. Brussels: Council of European Communities.

Council of European Communities (1977) Council Directive (77/452/EEC) concerning the mutual recognition of diplomas, certificates and other evidence of the formal qualifications of nurses responsible for general care, including measures to facilitate the effective exercise of this right of establishment and freedom to provide services.

Council of European Communities (1977) Council Directive (77/453/EEC) concerning the co-ordination of provisions laid down by law, regulation or administrative action in respect of the activities of nurses responsible for general care. Brussels: Council of European Communities.

Department of Finance (1997) *Commission on Public Service Pensions - Interim Report.*
Dublin: Stationary Office.

Department of Health and Children (1997) Report of the Working Group on the Role of the Mental Handicap Nurse (Unpublished).

Department of Health and Children (1997) Public Health Nursing - A Review (Unpublished).

Department of Health and Children (1997) *Commission on Nursing - Interim Report.*
Dublin: Stationary Office.

Department of Health (1997) *Enhancing the Partnership: Report of the Working Group on the Implementation of the Health Strategy in Relation to persons with Mental Handicap.*
Dublin: Department of Health.

Department of Health (1995) *Survey of Long-Stay Units 1994.* Dublin: Department of Health.

Department of Health (1994) *Shaping a Healthier Future, a strategy for effective health care in the 1990's.* Dublin: Department of Health.

Department of Health (1991) *Needs and Abilities:A Policy for the Intellectually Disabled: Report of the Review Group on Mental Handicap Services.* Dublin: Stationary Office.

Department of Health (1990) *Dublin Hospitals Initiative Group - Interim Report.*
Dublin: Department of Health.

Department of Health (1988) *The Years Ahead - A Policy for the Elderly.* Dublin: Stationary Office.

Department of Health (1984) *The Psychiatric Services - Planning for the Future:Report of a Study Group on the Development of the Psychiatric Services.* Dublin: Stationary Office.

Department of Health (1980) *Working Party on General Nursing Report,* Dublin: Stationary Office.

Department of Health (1966) Circular 27/66 on District Nursing Scheme.

Douglas, Robin (1998) Planning for Personal Development. *Office for Health Management* Issue 3, May.

European Council for Ministers (1996) *Council of Europe Recommendations on Nursing Research.* No. R(96)1, Brussels: Commission of the European Communities.

Hart, G. (1985) College-Based Education: Background and Bugs. *The Australian Nurses Journal* 15(4), 46-48.

Health Research Board (1997) *Annual Report of the National Intellectual Disability Database Committee* (1996). Dublin: Health Research Board.

Health Research Board (1996) *Annual Report and Accounts '96*. Dublin: Health Research Board.

International Council for Nurses (1992) *Guidelines on Specialisation in Nursing*. R(96)1, Brussels: Commission of the European Communities.

International Confederation of Midwives (ICM) (1972) *Definition of a midwife*, adopted by the ICM and by the International Federation of Gynaecology and Obstetrics (1973). Amended and ratified by the International Federation of Gynaecology and Obstetrics (1991) and the World Health Organisation (1992).

Irish Business and Employers Confederation (1998) Draft Guidelines on Bullying (Unpublished).

J.M. Consulting (1998) The Regulation of Nurses, Midwives and Health Visitors - invitation to Comment on Issues Raised by a Review of the Nurses, Midwives and Health Visitors Act 1997, Commissioned by the four UK Health Departments (Unpublished).

Labour Court (1997) Recommendation No. LRC 15450, CD/97/48.

Lewis, T. (1990) The Hospital Ward Sister: Professional Gate Keeper. *Journal of Advanced Nursing* 15, 808-818.

Lyons, R. Tivey, H. and Ball, C. Bullying at Work: How to Tackle it - A guide for MSF Representatives and Members of MSF Union (Unpublished).

National Council on Ageing and Older People (1997) *The Years Ahead Report: A Review of the Implementation of its Recommendations*. Dublin: National Council on Ageing and Older People.

Organisation for Economic Co-operation and Development (1997) *OECD Economic Survey, Ireland 1997*. Paris: OECD.

Price-Waterhouse (1997) Nursing Applications Centre - Review of Operations for the Department of Health and Children (Unpublished).

Price-Waterhouse (1997) Report on Project Management of the Nursing Applications Centre (NAC) for the Department of Health and Children (Unpublished).

Robertson, F. (1993) *Survey of Directors of Nursing and Employer Organisations and Comparisons with Students and Faculties of Ratings of Nursing Degree Programs*. Study Prepared for the National Review of Nurse Education in the Higher Education Sector, National Institute of Labour Studies, Flinders University and the University of Melbourne.

Royal College of Nursing (1997) The Future of Nurse Education. *Nursing Standard* 11(34) 22-24.

Royal College of Nursing (1994) *Must it be so Hard? Hardship Amongst Nurse Students*. London: RCN.

Royal College of Nursing (1988) *Specialities in Nursing*. London: RCN.

Russell, L. Gething, L. and Convery, P. (1997) *National Review of Specialist Nurse Education*. Canberra: Commonwealth of Australia.

Statute of the Council of Europe Article 15.b. in International Council for Nurses (1992) *Guidelines on Specialisation in Nursing. R(96)1, Brussels: Commission of the European Communities*.

Statutory Instrument 256 of 1996. Medicinal Products (Prescription and Control of Supply) Regulations, 1996.

United Kingdom Central Council for Nursing and Midwifery and Health Visiting (1996) *Guidelines for Professional Practice.* London: UKCC.

United Kingdom Central Council for Nursing and Midwifery and Health Visiting (1994) *The Council's Standards for Education and Practice Following Registration.* London: UKCC.

United Kingdom Central Council for Nursing and Midwifery and Health Visiting (1992) *The Scope of Professional Practice.* London: UKCC.

University of Newcastle, Central Coast Area Health Services and New South Wales Nurses Registration Board (1997) *Project to review and examine expectations of beginning registered nurses in the workforce.* Sydney: Nurses Registration Board of New South Wales.

World Health Organisation (1996) *Nursing Practice - Report of a WHO Expert Committee.* Geneva: World Health Organisation.

Acts

Freedom of Information Act 1997.

Child Care Act 1991.

Health (Nursing Homes) Act 1990.

Safety, Health and Welfare at Work Act 1989.

Data Protection Act 1988.

Nurses Act 1985.

Misuse of Drugs Act 1984.

Medical Practitioners Act 1978.

Misuse of Drugs Act 1977.

Health Act 1970.

Nurses Act 1943 (UK).

Bibliography (Chapter 2)

Barrington, R. (1979) *Health, Medicine and Politics in Ireland 1900-1970*.
Dublin: Institute of Public Administration.

Barry, J. (1992) *The Victoria Hospital, Cork: A History 1874-1986*. Cork.: Litho.

Burke, H. (1993) *The Royal Hospital Donnybrook: A Heritage of Caring 1743-1993*.
Dublin: Royal Hospital Donnybrook and the Social Science Research Centre, University College Dublin.

Coakley, D. (1992) *Doctor Steevens' Hospital: a brief history*. Dublin: Dr. Steevens' Hospital.

Coakley, D. (1988) *The Irish School of Medicine*. Dublin: Townhouse.

Farmar, T. (1994) *Holles Street 1894-1994*. Dublin: A & A Farmar.

Gatenby, P. (1996) *Dublin's Meath Hospital 1753-1996*. Dublin: Town House.

Henry, H.M. (1989) *Our Lady's Hospital, Cork - history of the mental hospital in Cork
spanning 200 years*. Cork: Haven Books.

Irish Nurses Organisation, (1969) *Fiftieth Anniversary Souvenir Book*. Dublin: INO.

Kirkpatrick, T. P. (1924) *The History of Dr. Steevens' Hospital 1720-1920*. Dublin: University Press.

Lyons, J.B. (1991) *The Quality of Mercers: The Story of Mercer's Hospital 1784-1991*.
Dublin: Glendale.

McCarthy, G. (1997) Nursing and the Health Services, in Robins, J. *Reflections on Health*.
Dublin: Institute of Public Administration.

Meenan F.O.C. (1972) *The Children's Hospital, Temple Street, Dublin - Centenary Book, 1872-1972*.
Dublin: Temple Street.

Meenan, F.O.C. (1995) *St Vincent's Hospital 1834-1994, an historical and social portrait*.
Dublin: Gill and MacMillan.

Moore, H. (1942) The Nursing Profession and its Needs. *Studies 31*.

Nolan, M. E.(1991) *One Hundred Years: A History of the School of Nursing and of developments
at the Mater Hospital 1891-1991*. Dublin: Mater Hospital.

O'Brien, E.; O'Malley, K and Browne, L. (1988) *The House of Industry Hospitals, 1772-1987:
The Richmond, Whitworth and Hardwicke (St. Laurence's Hospital): A Closing Menoir*.
Dublin: Anniversary Press.

O'Brien, E. (1987) *The Charitable Infirmary Jervis Street 1718-1987*, a Farewell Tribute.
Dublin: Anniversary Press.

O'Brien, E.; Crookshank, A. and Wolstenholne, G. (1984) *A Portrait of Irish Medicine:
An Illustrated History of Medicine in Ireland*. Dublin: Ward River Press.

Robins, J. (1995) *The Miasma: Epidemic and Panic in Nineteenth Century Ireland*.
Dublin: Institute of Public Administration.

Robins, J. (1995) Public Policy and the Maternity Services in, Browne, A.
Masters, Midwives and Ladies-in-Waiting. Dublin: A & A Farmar.

Robins, J. (1992) *From Rejection to Integration: A centenary of service by the Daughters of Charity to persons with mental handicap.* Dublin: Gill and Macmillan Ltd.

Scanlan, P, (1991) *The Irish Nurse: A Study of Nursing in Ireland.* Manorhamilton: Drumlin.

Walsh, D. (1997) Mental Care in Ireland 1945-1997 and the Future, in Robins, J. *Reflections on Health.* Dublin: Institute of Public Administration.

Widdess, J.D.H. (1984) *The Royal College of Surgeons in Ireland and its Medical School 1784-1984.* Dublin: Royal College of Surgeons in Ireland.

Widdess, J.D.H. (1972) *The Richmond, Whitworth, Hardwicke Hospitals, St Laurences Dublin, 1772-1972.* Dublin.

Wiley, M. (1997) Financing the Irish Health Services in Robins, J. *Reflections on Health.* Dublin: Institute of Public Administration.

Woodham - Smith, C. (1950) *Florence Nightingale 1820-1910.* London: Constable.

1. Ms. Liz Sheridan
    Co. Sligo

2. A McCarthy
    Co. Cork

3. Ms. Noreen Roche
    Co. Tipperary

4. Ms. Catherine Hayes
    London

5. Anonymous

6. Nurses
    St. Joseph's Hospital
    Castletownbere
    Co. Cork

7. Mr. Martin Clancy
    Co. Clare

8. Ms. Kay Shine
    Co. Louth

9. Ms. Clare Kelly
    National Children's Hospital
    Dublin 2

10. Staff Nurses
    Macroom District Hospital

11. Mr. Gearoid Donnchadha
    Co. Wicklow

12. Assistant Nurses
    St. John of God Brothers
    Co. Louth

13. Ms. Maureen Gaughran
    Co. Louth

14. Nursing Staff
    St. Camillus' Hospital
    Limerick

15. Ms. Breda Brady
    Dublin 2

16. Ms. Claire Nee

17. Mr. Malachy Feely
    Co. Meath

18. Ms. Orla Ryan
    Dublin 18

19. Mr. John O'Neill
    Co. Wexford

20. Ms. Catherine Hogan
    Dublin 14

21. Ms. Erica Shipman
    Co. Dublin

22. Mrs. Kathleen Ensko
    Co. Mayo

23. "A Service without Walls" -
    An Analysis of Public Health
    Nursing in 1994

24. Mr. Martin Hewitt
    Co. Kildare

25. Mrs. Anne Forde
    Co. Offaly

26. Ms. Margaret Walshe
    Dublin 15

27. Ms. Sheila O'Connor
    Co. Cork

28. Public Health Nurses
    in North Kerry

29. Staff Working in three Psychiatric
    Day Centres Eastern Health Board

30. Public Health Nurses
    Dublin 9

31. Ms. Clara Ni Ghiolla
    Belfast

32. Mr. Donal O'Sullivan
    & Mr. Winifred Leonard
    Dublin 7

33. Mr. Liam Gormley
    Co. Wicklow

34. Hospital Pharmacists' Association
    Ireland

35. Mr. Jimmy Stenson
    Co. Westmeath

36. M Finlay
Co. Laois

37. Anonymous

38. Ms. Teresa Lynch
Co. Laois

39. Anonymous

40. Ms. Brigid O'Connor
Co. Cork

41. Ms. Ursula Cafferty
Co. Westmeath

42. Ms. Betty Foley
Co. Kerry

43. Ms. Mary Kelly
Co. Kerry

44. Ms. Mary Teresa Devane
Co. Kerry

45. Nursing Administration
General Hospital Tullamore

46. Ms. Marie Conlon
Co. Laois

47. Temporary Nursing Staff
Co. Laois

48. Representation of Staff from a
Day Activity Centre for People
with Learning Disabilities in Dublin

49. Enrolled Nurses
Cherry Orchard Hospital

50. Institute of Guidance Counsellors
North Eastern Branch
Co. Monaghan

51. Ms. Ann Winters
Co. Mayo

52. Ms. Colette Costello
Limerick

53. Ms. Eithne O'Reilly Gulry
Cavan

54. Ms. Catherine Hanrahan
Limerick

55. Ms. Claire Crowe
Dublin 12

56. Mr. Brian Denham
Dublin 4

57. Irish Association of Nursing
in Aids Care (IANAC)

58. Ms. Anne McElligott
Co. Kerry

59. Ms. Helen Duffy
Co. Dublin

60. Ms. Margaret Cotter
Co. Cork

61. Ms. Eileen Hennigan
Co. Dublin

62. Ms. Fionnuala O'Gorman
Cork

63. Detoxification Unit
Beaumont Hospital

64. Home Care Management Team
From Swords & Balbriggan
Co. Dublin

65. Mr. Albert Murphy
Waterford

66. Ms. Mary Thornton
Co. Clare

67. Ms. Patricia Lynch Manning
Co. Cork

68. Ms. Bernadette Walker
Co. Westmeath

69. Ms. Veronica Gibbons
Co. Westmeath

70. Ms. Rose Conlon
Co. Westmeath

71. Ms. Pauline Woods
Co. Louth

72. Longford Public Health Nurses

73. Mrs. Phil Yourell
Co. Westmeath

74. Mrs. Theresa Maguire
Dublin 9

75. Nurse Tutors
Co. Donegal

76. Mr. Tony Barden
Waterford

77. Pat O'Neill
Waterford

78. Mr. Tom Clare
Dublin 14

79. Sunbeam House Services
Co. Wicklow

80. Ms. Valarie Small
Dublin 8

81. Midwifery Tutors from the
Midwifery Training Schools

82. Mr. William Cronin
Cork

83. Senior Public Health Nurses
South Eastern Health Board

84. Ms. Geraldine Darcy
Limerick

85. Night Sisters
COPE Foundation
Cork

86. Ms. Nora Quill
Co. Cork

87. Student Midwives
Co. Cork

88. Ms. Monica M Collins
Co. Offaly

89. Nursing Staff Involved in Care of
the Elderly Midland Health Board

90. Ms. Mary Dunne
Co. Offaly

91. Acute Pain Service
Beaumont Hospital

92. Nursing Advisory Forum of the
Irish Association for Palliative Care

93. Nurses/Addiction Counsellors
Western Health Board

94. Mr. Joe Faulkner
Sligo General Hospital

95. Ms. Catherine O'Sullivan
Cork

96. Theatre Department
Waterford Regional Hospital

97. Nursing Staff
St. Brendan's Home, Co. Galway

98. Staff Nurses
Brothers of Charity Services
Boyle

99. Ms. Ann Sharkey
Co. Louth

100. Ms. Sheila O'Reilly
Cork

101. Nurse Manager Branch
Psychiatric Nurses Association

102. Ms. Philomena Stynes
Co. Dublin

103. Unit Nurse Officers/Services Managers
Sligo General Hospital

104. Ms. Margo Topham
Cork

105. Nurse Tutors
Letterkenny

106. Nurses from Carrigoran
Nursing Home
Co. Clare

107. Ms. Mary Kelly
Co. Offaly

108. Ms. Maureen Crowley
Co. Cork

109. Nursing Administrator Sisters
in Beaumont Hospital in Charge
of Out of Hours Services

110. Community Psychiatric Nurses
Sligo

111. Mr. Henry Abbott
Co. Westmeath

112. Staff from the Outpatient Department
St. John's Hospital
Limerick

113. Phil Murphy
Co. Cork

114. Community Nurses working
within Early Childhood Services
in the Brothers of Charity in
Galway and Roscommon

115. Rehab Unit
St. Mary's Hospital
Mullingar

116. J Leahy
Kilkenny

117. Ms. Nora Garahy
Co. Offaly

118. First Floor Staff Nurses
St. John's Hospital
Limerick

119. Ms. Judith Chavasse
Dublin 14

120. Infection Control Nurses
Association (Irish Group)

121. Nurses working in the Eastern
Health Board's Aids/Drugs Services

122. The Donegal Practice Nurses

123. Psychiatric Nurses with Family
Therapy Qualifications from
North Western Health Board

124. Community Nursing Group
Area 7 Psychiatric Services
Eastern Health Board

125. Community Psychiatric Nurses
in the Roscommon Psychiatric Service

126. Sligo Association of Critical
Care Nurses (S.A.C.C.N.)

127. Ms. M O'Flynn
Co. Cork

128. Ms. Elaine O'Dwyer
Waterford Regional Hospital

129. Ms. Frances McHugh
Sligo General Hospital

130. Public Health Nurses Institute
of Community Health Nursing
Longford/Westmeath Branch

131. Representative Group of Nurses
working in New and Developing
Community Mental Health Projects
in the Mayo Psychiatric Service

132. INO Members
District Hospital
Listowel

133. 3rd Year Students (1994 Intake)
Letterkenny General Hospital

134. Nurses from
COPE Foundation
Cork

135. Ms. Mary Syron
Co. Galway

136. Ms. Helen Plunkett
Limerick

137. Anonymous

138. Ms. Anna O'Brien
Cork

139. Anonymous

140. Regional Technical Colleges
Nurses

141. Mr. Eugene Caulfield
North Eastern Health Board

142. Ms. Eilis Fullam
Co. Kildare

143. Ms. Deirdre Clarke
Dublin 5

144. Ms. Rita Moloney
Co. Kildare

145. L Kelly
Dublin 14

146. Ms. Jane Donohue
Co. Meath

147. Public Health Nurses
Tuam, Co. Galway

148. Ms. Mary Glennon
Co. Kildare

149. Ward Sisters employed
by COPE Foundation, Cork

150. Nurses engaged in the Addiction
Service for the Elderly at Cork
University/St. Finbarr's Hospitals

151. Senior Public Health Nurses
Institute of Community
Health Nursing

152. Psychiatric Nurse Managers
in the Cork Area

153. Clinical Nurse Specialist Group
in Cystic Fibrosis in Ireland

154. Midwifery Staff
National Maternity Hospital

155. Nursing Staff
Portiuncula Hospital
Galway

156. Mr. Lawrence Cunningham
Co. Westmeath

157. Ms. Eileen Fitzgerald
Kilkenny

158. Ms. Margaret O'Connell
Waterford

159. Ms. Bridget Ryan
Co. Cork

160. Staff from the Intensive Care Unit
Wexford General Hospital

161. Ms. Patricia F Harte
Sligo General Hospital

162. The Nurses of St. Columbanus Home
Killarney

163. Ms. Mary Burke
Co. Tipperary

164. Irish Association of Counsellors
Midland Health Board Regional Group

165. Mr. Michael O'Keeffe
Co. Cork

166. Ms. Mary Mulvihill
Co. Tipperary

167. Community Psychiatric Nurses
East Galway Psychiatric Services

168. Ms. Marie McCarthy
Co. Cork

169. Ms. Marion Moriarty
Limerick

170. Ms. Myriam Leahy
Co. Cork

171. Anonymous

172. Irish Nursing Research
Interest Group

173. Matrons' of the Geriatric
Hospitals of the South East Region

174. Nursing Officers in the
Mayo Psychiatric Services

175. Staff Nurses
Coronary Care Unit
Beaumont Hospital

176. Ms. Rita Smith
Dublin 16

177. Ms. Anne Fox
Dublin 9

178. Ms. Maura O'Brien
Co. Tipperary

179. Ms. Frances Kennedy
Co. Tipperary

180. Ms. Moya Carroll
Cavan

181. Community Psychiatric
Nurses from the South Eastern
Health Board

182. Diabetes Nurses
Beaumont Hospital

183. Ms. Margaret McCarthy
Limerick Regional Hospital

184. Senior Public Health Nurses
Co. Kerry

185. Mr. Jim Thomas
Co. Mayo

186. Irish Association of
Critical Care Nurses

187. St. Colman's Hospital
Co. Wicklow

188. Members of Institute of
Community Health Nursing

189. Generic Community Psychiatric
Nurses in the Donegal Area of the
North Western Health Board

190. Senior Nurse Managers
South Eastern Health Board

191. Ms. Deirdre Kavanagh
& Ms. Maura Colgan
Eastern Health Board

192. Nurse Tutors
School of Nursing
Sligo

193. Ms. Ita Tighe
Dublin 3

194. The Cognitive
Behavioural Psychotherapists
North Western Health Board

195. Community Psychiatric Clinical
Nurse Specialists in Addiction
in the Donegal Area of the
North Western Health Board

196. Association of Administrative
Psychiatric Nurses (AAPN)

197. Ms. Marianne Doran
Beaumont Hospital

198. Staff Nurses
Top Floor, St. John's Hospital
Limerick

199. Public Health Nurses
Mid-Western Health Board

200. Liver Transplant Co-ordinators
St. Vincent's Hospital
Dublin 4

201. Nursing Officer Group (Psych)
St. Loman's Hospital
Dublin 20

202. Education Committee
St. Loman's Hospital
Dublin 20

203. Public Health Nurses
Class 96/97
University College Dublin

204. Course Co-ordinators
St. Vincent's/Mater Hospitals

205. Ms. Sandy Mason
Co. Louth

206. Ms. Noreen Keane
Dublin 9

207. Ms. Eileen McKenna
Co. Kerry

208. Ms. Sinead Hanafin
University College Cork

209. Mr. Mark Monahan
Dublin 9

210. Ms. Martina Kehoe
Waterford Regional Hospital

211. Ms. Joan Phyllis Kirwan
Waterford Regional Hospital

212. Ms. Susan O'Donoghue
Waterford Regional Hospital

213. Dr. Colin Buckley
Waterford Regional Hospital

214. Ms. Avril O'Leary
Dublin 9

215. Mr. Jim Brosnan
Dublin 20

216. Nurse Members attached
to Clondalkin and Tallaght
Mental Health Services
from St. Loman's Hospital
Dublin 20

217. Mr. Malachy Nugent
Dublin 7

218. Ms. Mary Tynan

219. Theatre Nursing Staff
Beaumont Hospital

220. Ms. Siobhan Ní Scanaill
& Ms. Jane Leavy
Dublin 8

References, Bibliography, Appendices and Acknowledgements

221. Members of the Irish Association of Operating Theatre Superintendents/Managers

222. Director and Family Development Nurses of the Community Mothers Programme Eastern Health Board

223. Saville & Holdsworth University of Limerick

224. Nurse Education Committee Sligo General Hospital

225. Diabetes Nurse Specialist Group St. Vincent's Hospital Dublin 4

226. Department of Community Psychiatric Nursing St. Patrick's Hospital Dublin 8

227. Community RGNs Dublin 14

228. Renal Unit Sligo General Hospital

229. Ms. Bernie Morrisroe Sligo General Hospital

230. Ms. Mary Gillan Sligo General Hospital

231. Ms. Madeleine Munnelly Sligo General Hospital

232. L Ruttledge Sligo General Hospital

233. Ms. Noreen O'Sullivan Sligo General Hospital

234. Ms. Mary Flatley Sligo General Hospital

235. Ms. Karen Reynolds Sligo General Hospital

236. Ms. Margaret Towey Sligo General Hospital

237. G O'Brien Sligo General Hospital

238. Ms. Karen E Fagan Sligo General Hospital

239. Ms. Maureen Campbell Sligo General Hospital

240. Ms. Rosemary Irwin Sligo General Hospital

241. Ms. Ciara Swayelen Sligo General Hospital

242. Staff Nurses working in the Field of Learning Disabilities Cork

243. Ms. Imelda B McCarthy Cork

244. Ms. Joan Phelan

245. Midwifery Staff Rotunda Hospital

246. Public Health Nurses Southern Health Board

247. Ms. Margaret Freeney Limerick

248. Public Health Nurses Roscommon Area

249. Junior Ward Sisters Intensive Care Unit Beaumont Hospital

250. Staff Nurses Intensive Care Unit Beaumont Hospital

251. Ms. Sheila Fitzgerald Dublin 10

252. Ms. Mary Villiers Co. Cork

253. Ms. Elizabeth Doyle Dublin 15

254. Ms. Patricia Campbell Co. Meath

255. Public Health Nurses/ Addiction Counsellors Eastern Health Board

256. Nursing Staff Ard Aoibhinn Centre Wexford

References, Bibliography, Appendices and Acknowledgements

257. Lifford Community Hospital

258. Dual Qualified Registered Psychiatric
     and Registered General Nurses
     Tralee General Hospital

259. Ms. Caroline Dolan &
     Ms. Catherine Croffy
     Co. Galway

260. Terry Hayes
     Co. Waterford

261. National University of Ireland - Galway

262. Theatre Staff
     Lourdes Orthopaedic Hospital
     Kilkenny

263. Nursing Staff
     Lourdes Orthopaedic Hospital
     Kilkenny

264. INO Midwife Members
     The Coombe Hospital
     Dublin 8

265. Ms. Maureen Lynn
     & Ms. Jacqueline Egan
     Dublin 8

266. St. Vincent's Hospital
     Fairview
     Dublin 3

267. Health Counsel
     Dublin 3

268. Nursing Staff
     St. Patrick's Ward
     Beaumont Hospital

269. Ms. Angela Lally
     Dublin Dental Hospital

270. Health Sciences Group
     of the Library Association of Ireland

271. Ms. Margaret O'Brien
     Dublin 6

272. Ms. Anne Murphy
     Meath Hospital
     & Ms. Anna Craig
     National Children's Hospital

273. Irish Pharmaceutical Union

274. Ms. Sandra Keating
     Co. Offaly

275. Ms. Mary Riordan
     Dublin 2

276. Irish Business and
     Employers Confederation

277. Tutorial Staff
     School of Nursing, Mater Hospital

278. Liaison Nurses Forum
     Our Lady's Hospital for Sick Children
     Crumlin

279. Director of Nursing and Nursing Staff
     from The Children's Hospital
     Temple Street

280. Anonymous

281. Nurses from
     Phlebotomy, Urodynamics
     and Outpatient Departments
     Beaumont Hospital

282. Ms. Edwina O'Keeffe
     Kilkenny

283. Occupational Health Department
     Waterford Regional Hospital

284. Nursing Staff
     St. Patrick's Geriatric Hospital
     Cashel, Co. Tipperary

285. National Nursing
     Sisters Association

286. Midwives in Ultrasonography
     Rotunda Hospital

287. Maternity Unit
     Letterkenny General Hospital

288. Cork Voluntary Hospitals
     School of Nursing

289. Ms. Eileen Cullen
     & Ms. Eilis Breen

290. Ms. Marguerite McGilly Cuddy
     Wexford

291. Female Surgical
     St. Luke's General Hospital, Kilkenny

292. Ms. Una Webster
Co. Cork

293. Mr. Sean McCarty
Waterford

294. Ms. Marie Healy
Co. Cork

295. RNMH's working in the
community in Cork and Kerry

296. Ms. Maureen Cahill
Co. Cork

297. Ms. Maura Fagan
Co. Louth

298. Matrons/Directors of Nursing
Care of the Elderly Service
North Eastern Health Board

299. Area Co-ordinators
Care of the Elderly
North Eastern Health Board

300. The Irish Matrons' Association

301. Psychiatric Nurses
Area 7 Psychiatric Services
Eastern Health Board

302. The National Rehabilitation Hospital
Dun Laoghaire

303. A Fitzsimons
Royal Victoria Eye and Ear Hospital
Dublin 2

304. Ms. Breda Jones
Dublin 3

305. Institute of Public Administration

306. Mrs. Eileen Maher
& Ms. Wendy Fair
St. Luke's Hospital
Dublin 6

307. Faculty of Health Sciences
Trinity College Dublin

308. Union of Students in Ireland

309. M W Quigley
Galway

310. Domiciliary Midwives and
Home Births in Ireland

311. National Rehabilitation Board

312. Association of Nurse Teachers

313. Mr. John Fitzpatrick
Co. Kildare

314. Ms. Patricia Fitzpatrick
Co. Kildare

315. Ward Sister Association
St. Finbarr's Hospital, Cork

316. Ms. Jean Harrison
North Eastern Health Board
Harcourt Street

317. Ward Sisters
St. Luke's Hospital, Kilkenny

318. Public Health Nurses
Area 2, Eastern Health Board

319. Mr. Geoff Day
North Eastern Health Board

320. Ms. Jane Boyle
Donegal

321. Ms. Clare O'Herlihy
Cork

322. Nurses from St. Anne's Hospital
Dublin 6

323. National Neurosurgical Unit
Beaumont Hospital

324. The Board
Faculty of Nursing
Royal College of Surgeons in Ireland

325. Outreach Counsellors working
in the Aids/Drugs Service of the
Eastern Health Board

326. Nursing Staff of the Adelaide and
Meath Hospital incorporating
the National Children's Hospital

327. Nursing Staff
St. Loman's Hospital, Mullingar

328. Nursing School
National Children's Hospital
Harcourt Street

329. Nursing Staff of the
National Children's Hospital

330. Cardiac Catheterization Laboratory
St. James's Hospital

331. Radiology Staff Nurses
St. James's Hospital

332. Behaviour Nurse Psychotherapists
from the Eastern Region

333. Ms. Miriam McCarthy
Co. Wicklow

334. B N Brown
Galway

335. National Senior Public
Health Nurses

336. Senior Public Health Nurses
of the Eastern Health Board

337. The Irish Association for
Nurses in Oncology

338. Ms. Joan Kelly
Irish Cancer Society

339. Midwives
Our Lady of Lourdes Hospital,
Drogheda

340. Nursing and Midwifery Staff
Our Lady of Lourdes Hospital,
Drogheda

341. Nurse Tutors
School of Nursing, Beaumont Hospital

342. Mr. Martin Connor
& Mr. John McTiernan
Community Care Area 8
Eastern Health Board

343. Nursing Administration
and Nursing Staff
St. Vincent's Hospital
Co. Laois

344. Ms. Lorna Kelleher
Cork

345. The Nurse Teachers
The School of Nursing
St. Vincent's Hospital
Elm Park, Dublin 4

346. Miss J Bartley
Beaumont Hospital

347. Psychiatric Nurse Managers
in the Cork area

348. Irish Registered Nursing
Homes Association

349. Department of Nursing
St. Vincent's Hospital
Elm Park, Dublin 4

350. Ms. Joan Moyles
Co. Mayo

351. The National Superintendent
Public Health Nurses Group

352. Ms. Joan Murray
Beaumont Hospital

353. Association of Family Planning
Nurses Ireland

354. Dr. Aine O'Sullivan
Cavan

355. Staff Nurses
COPE Foundation
Hollyhill, Cork

356. Senior Nurse Managers
St. Finbarr's Hospital
Cork

357. Public Health Students
National University of Ireland - Cork

358. Nursing Staff
Medical Floor
St. Luke's Hospital
Kilkenny

359. Ms. Margaret Maguire
Sligo General Hospital

360. Mr. John McNally
Monaghan

361. St. Bridget's Hospital
Carrick-on-Suir
Co. Tipperary

362. Ms. Noreen Cremin
Co. Kerry

363. Community Psychiatric Nurses
Community Care Area 8
Eastern Health Board

364. Board and Staff of
Cheeverstown House Limited
Templeogue
Dublin 6W

365. Ms. Irene O'Mahony
& Ms. Karen Kelleher
National University of Ireland - Cork

366. Ms. Mary Burke
Co. Offaly

367. Ms. Ciara Davin
Dublin 4

368. Group of West Cork
Public Health Nurses

369. Nursing Staff
St. John's Community Hospital
Sligo

370. Ms. Breda O'Donoghue
Co. Cork

371. Staff from
St. Patrick's Hospital
Cashel, Co. Tipperary

372. Ms. Brigid Caldwell
Co. Longford

373. Ms. Norma Kissane
Co. Kerry

374. Anonymous

375. Ms. Stephanie Ryan
Co. Tipperary

376. Ms. Mary Cullinan
Co. Offaly

377. Ms. Ann Cahalane
Co. Cork

378. Ms. Marion Barnes
Co. Kerry

379. Mr. David Healy,
Co. Cork

380. Ms. Kathryn Healy,
Co. Cork

381. Ms. Sarah A Lawless
Co. Mayo

382. Ms. Helen P McLoughlin
Co. Offaly

383. Ms. Fiona Robins-Claffey
Co. Offaly

384. Ms. Eileen O'Heney
Co. Westmeath

385. Ms. Peggy Murtagh
Co. Westmeath

386. Nurses
Eye Department
Waterford Regional Hospital

387. Ms. Elizabeth Cuddy Devine
Roscommon

388. Ms. Nuala Cashlin
Letterkenny General Hospital
& Ms. Ann Monaghan
Sligo General Hospital

389. Ms. Jill Anthony
Waterford Regional Hospital

390. Accident & Emergency Sisters
Beaumont Hospital

391. Geriatric Section
Sacred Heart Hospital, Castlebar

392. Ms. Maura Walsh
Waterford Regional Hospital

393. Senior Nurse Managers
Donegal Mental Health Services

394. Ward Sisters & Junior Ward Sisters
Brothers of Charity
Co. Roscommon Services

395. Ward Sisters
Sligo General Hospital

396. Registered Nurses in Mental Handicap
St. Vincent's Centre, Co. Limerick

397. Rescue Trust

398. Degree Nurses Association

399. Dermatologist Nurses
City of Dublin Skin and
Cancer Hospital
Dublin 2

400. Working Group
National Association for the
Mentally Handicapped of Ireland

401. Stoma Care Department
Baggot Street Community Hospital

402. October 1996 intake of Student
Nurses at Sligo General Hospital

403. Registered General Nurses in
Community Care Area 4
who are Members of IMPACT

404. Mr. Paul Gallagher
Dublin 9

405. Ms. Bernadette Carpenter
Co. Dublin

406. Nursing Staff
Heath County Infirmary
Navan

407. Ms. Maria M Murphy
Cork

408. Ms. Ann Mason
Cork

409. Ms. Triona Leyden
Co. Sligo

410. Anonymous

411. Ms. Dolores Gavin Doyle
Co. Cork

412. Ms. Ellen Manny
Co. Westmeath

413. St. Luke's Hospital
Kilkenny

414. Ms. Eleanor O'Connor
Cork

415. Anonymous

416. Ms. Kathleen McGovern
Sligo

417. Unit Directors of the Galway
County Association for
Mentally Handicapped Children

418. Ms. Margaret Dillon
Limerick

419. Association of Behaviour
Therapists in Services for
People with Learning Disabilities

420. Ms. Claire Gough
Co. Mayo

421. SIPTU Members
Mayo Health Services

422. Bed Managers Group
St. James's Hospital

423. St. Brigid's CPN Group
Co. Louth

424. Louth/Meath Family
Therapy Service

425. Ms. Geraldine Hoyne
Co. Tipperary

426. Mr. Eugene McCormack
Co. Mayo

427. Clinical Placement Co-ordinators
Beaumont Hospital

428. Ms. Catherine Lavin
& Ms. Mary O'Dowd
Co. Mayo

429. Tutorial Staff of
St. Louise's School of Nursing,
St. Joseph's Hospital
Dublin 15

430. Ward Sisters
Mater Misericordiae Hospital

431. Nursing Sisters
University College Hospital, Galway

432. Nurses
University College Hospital, Galway

433. Ms. Imelda Tobin
Co. Cork

434. Department of Nursing Studies
National University of Ireland - Dublin

435. Ms. Maureen Flynn
Dublin 4

436. Nursing Staff
Our Lady's Hospital for Sick Children
Crumlin

437. Nurse Managers Association
(Mental Handicap)

438. Association of Nurses in Radiology

439. Co-ordinators for Continuing
Education in three Health Board Areas

440. Ms. Catherine Quinn
Limerick

441. Mr. Oliver O'Connor
Cavan

442. Ms. Margaret Fleming
Monaghan

443. Ms. Imelda Connolly O'Connor
Co. Limerick

444. Ms. Lynda Moore
Cork

445. Ms. Mary Harvey
Co. Clare

446. Education Committee
Letterkenny General Hospital

447. Pat Monaghan
Galway

448. Nursing Officers and
Deputy Nursing Officers
St. Dympna's Hospital
Carlow

449. Computer Nurse Co-ordinators
Meath and Adelaide Hospitals

450. Ms. Mary Harte
Sligo General Hospital

451. The Irish Innovative Nurse
Management Network

452. Ms. Mary Kearney
Co. Galway

453. Ms. Maria McInerney
Limerick

454. Mr. Michael Gilligan,
Mr. Peadar Ryan
& Mr. Eugene McCormack

455. INO Members
St. John's Hospital
Enniscorthy

456. Ms. Marian Keely
Co. Tipperary

457. Ms. Sheila Reilly
Co. Tipperary

458. Ward Sisters
University College Hospital
Galway

459. Chief Nursing Officer Group
(Psychiatric Service)
Eastern Health Board

460. Nursing Staff
University College Hospital
Galway

461. Public Health Nurses
in Community Care Area 5
Eastern Health Board

462. Ms. Veronica Mee
Co. Dublin

463. Dr. Colette Halpin
on behalf of Child
Psychiatrists in Ireland

464. Nurse Management
Limerick Regional Hospital

465. Mr. David Kieran
Co. Tipperary

466. Ms. Rita Higgins
Cavan

467. Educational Committee
Mallow General Hospital

468. Ms. Kathleen Seaver
Kilkenny

469. Cork and Kerry Nurse
Education Committee

470. Louth/Meath Hospital Group

471. Ms. Mary Rogers
Galway

472. Ms. Anne O'Byrne
Co. Wicklow

473. St. Angela's College of Education
Sligo

474. Professor John Carroll
Dublin City University

475. Public Health Nurses
in the Gorey Area
Co. Wexford

476. Ms. Ita Healy
Co. Meath

477. Ms. Patricia Barrett
Co. Mayo

478. Mr. John Fennessy
Co. Tipperary

479. Night Superintendents
St. James's Hospital
St. Brigid's Hospital
Ballinasloe

480. Council of the Pharmaceutical
Nurses Society of Ireland
Cork

481. Public Health Nurses
Working Group
Cavan

482. Mr. John Murray
Waterford

483. Ms. Fiona McGrath
Dublin 7

484. Ms. Mary Doyle
Wexford General Hospital

485. Ms. Nora Kane
Waterford Regional Hospital
Co. Roscommon

486. Ms. Mary Heffernan
Co. Limerick

487. Ms. Anne Costigan
Tipperary

488. Ms. Ann Gallagher
Co. Donegal

489. Ms. Joan Meaney
Limerick

490. Ms. Anne Gilbourne
Limerick Regional Hospital

491. Ms. Brigid Burke
Co. Waterford

492. Dialysis Unit
Letterkenny General Hospital

493. Nursing Officers & Deputy
Nursing Officers

494. Radiology/Cardiology
University College Hospital, Cork

495. Mr. Jim Brett
Co. Mayo

496. Ward Sisters & Staff Nurses
St. Nessan's Regional
Orthopaedic Hospital
Croom

497. Mr. Edmond McManamon
Co. Westmeath

498. Mr. Padraic Noone
Co. Galway

499. Ms. Mary Lyons
& Ms. Eileen Higgins
Co. Roscommon

500. Sisters of La Sagesse Services
Cregg House
Sligo

501. Nursing Staff
Intensive Care Unit
University College Hospital
Galway

502. Ms. Myra O'Brien
Co. Roscommon

503. Anonymous

504. Anonymous

505. Ms. Trina Nolan
Galway

506. Ms. Geraldine Flynn
Wexford General Hospital

507. Phil Mahony
Kilkenny

508. Mr. Barry Walsh
Carlow

509. Ms. Julia B Moloney
Co. Galway

510. State Enrolled Nurses working
in Hospitals in the Midlands

511. Ms. Sarah White
Co. Dublin

512. Mr. Peter Ledden
Dublin 3

513. Nursing Practice Development
Co-ordinators

514. Ms. Teresa Walsh
Galway

515. Ms. Deirdre Harrington
Co. Roscommon

516. Matrons of the Eastern
Health Board

517. Director of Nursing
and Nursing Staff
St. James's Hospital

518. Ms. Marie Molan
Co. Tipperary

519. Ward Sisters
General Hospital
Naas

520. Ms. Anne Cleary

521. Ms. Maeve Hanley,
Ms. Maureen Merne
& Ms. Teresa Murphy
Carlow

522. Ms. Anne Clarke
Co. Wicklow

523. Ms. Mary Durkin
Sligo General Hospital

524. Mr. P Finnegan
Co. Mayo

525. Ms. Sheena Faulkner

526. Ms. Olive Veerkamp
Co. Louth

527. Ms. Fiona Byrne

528. D Coyle
Co. Louth

529. Ms. Geraldine O'Reilly
Co. Louth

530. Ms. Ann McKenna
Co. Louth

531. Ms. Lorraine Glynn
Co. Louth

532. Ms. Antoinette Martin
Co. Louth

533. Ms. Geraldine Roche
Co. Louth

534. Lee Byrne
Co. Louth

535. Ms. Marian Spelman
Co. Louth

536. Ms. Aine McKenny
Co. Louth

537. Ms. Margaret Rowan
Co. Louth

538. Ms. Mary Cuthbert
Co. Louth

539. Ms. Stephanie Brennan
Co. Louth

540. Anonymous
Co. Limerick

541. Ms. Muriel Dawe
Co. Louth

542. Ms. Laura Breen
Co. Louth

543. Ms. Mary Courtney McDonnell
Co. Louth

544. Ms. Amanda Lavery
Co. Louth

545. Ms. Cathy Baylon
Co. Louth

546. Health and Safety Authority

547. Midwives Association of Ireland

548. Ms. Katherine Hogan
Waterford Regional Hospital

549. Sr. Nora Leonard
Co. Waterford

550. Ms. Alice O'Connor
Waterford

551. Mr. Eugene Cadden
Dublin 7

552. Ms. Margaret McCafferty
Sligo General Hospital

553. St. Louise's School of Nursing in
conjunction with Nurse Practitioners
from St. Joseph's Hospital
Dublin 15

554. Mrs. Brigid Barron
Co. Clare

555. Roscommon County Hospital

556. Ms. Lillian O'Connor
Co. Limerick

557. Ms. Deirdre Carroll
Co. Limerick

558. Mr. Gerard O'Neill
Waterford

559. School of Nursing
Waterford Regional Hospital

560. A Twomey
Waterford

561. The Federation of Voluntary Bodies
Galway Association

562. Mr. Willie Hackett
& Mr. Paul Maher

563. National University of Ireland
Nursing Studies Department

564. Ward Sisters
Tralee General Hospital

565. Ms. Alice Cox
Carlow

566. Phlebotomists Association of Ireland

567. Nursing Staff
St. Mary's Hospital
Dublin 20

568. Leslie Proudfoot
Dublin 4

569. Sr. Mary Morrisroe
Limerick

570. Ms. Elizabeth Heffernan
Co. Kerry

571. SIPTU Branch
St. Canice's Hospital
Kilkenny

572. Ms. Hannah O'Leary
Co. Tipperary

573. Ms. Cathy Kinsella
Kilkenny

574. Tutorial Staff, School of Nursing
Limerick Regional Hospital

575. Hospitaller Order of
Saint John of God
Co. Dublin

576. Ms. Angela Clarke
Co. Louth

577. Mid-Western Branch
Irish Nursing Research Interest Group

578. Nurse Managers/Matrons
Western Health Board Area

579. Ms. Annette Gee
Waterford Regional Hospital

580. The Nursing Staff of
Eastern Health Board
Child Psychiatric Services

581. Age and Opportunity
Marino Institute of Education
Dublin 9

582. Midwives
St. Finbarr's Hospital
Cork

583. Irish Health Services
Management Institute

584. Public Health Nurses
Community Care Area 4
Eastern Health Board

585. Ms. Bridget Kinsella
Co. Wicklow

586. Anonymous

587. Ward Attendants
Limerick Regional Hospital

588. Anonymous

589. Ms. Mary E Doherty
Co. Donegal

590. Public Health Nurses
New Ross Area

591. Ms. Mary Keogh
Carlow/Kilkenny

592. South Tipperary
Nursing Branch SIPTU

593. Ms. Teresa O'Brien
Co. Tipperary

594. Ms. Bridie O'Connor
Co. Galway

595. Ms. Mary Cronin
& Ms. Elke Hasner
North Eastern Health Board

596. Ms. Mary Killeen McCarthy
Co. Clare

597. Irish Practices Nurses Association
Kilkenny

598. Night Superintendents
North Eastern Health Board

599. Clinical Nurse Specialists
Eastern Health Board

600. Ms. Maura Ryan
Limerick

601. Mr. Michael O'Sullivan
Southern Health Board

602. Sr. Celestine
Co. Cork

603. Degree Nurses
Class of 1996
University College Cork

604. Matrons in Care of the Elderly
Mid-Western Health Board Area

605. Ms. Geraldine Freeman
Co. Galway

606. Public Health Nurses
Dingle Area

607. Care of the Elderly Day Hospital

608. School of Nursing
Tralee General Hospital

609. Staff Nurses
Tralee General Hospital

610. Public Health Nurses
of Co. Meath

611. Ms. Rena English
Co. Tipperary

612. Mr. Michael Bergin
Kilkenny

613. Ms. Christina Lambert
Co. Wexford

614. Behavioural Nurse Psychotherapists
North Eastern Health Board
Psychiatric Services

615. Palliative Care Team
Co. Monaghan

616. Mr. Liam Noud
Carlow

617. Ms. Margot Hanley
Limerick Regional Hospital

618. Ward Sisters
Limerick Regional Hospital

619. RNMH's
Early Childhood Services
Brothers of Charity
Co. Galway

620. Staff of Aras Attracta
Swinford
Co. Mayo

621. Staff of St. Mary's Day Hospital
Block 7
Orthopaedic Hospital
Cork

622. Ms. Rita Bourke
Galway

623. Control & Restraint Team
North Eastern Health Board

624. Ms. Agnes O'Sullivan
Co. Cork

625. National Superintendent
Public Health Management
Group Representing all
Health Boards

626. Nursing Officer & Deputy
Nursing Officers
Middleton

627. Staff from Cavan Day Hospital

628. SIPTU Members of CPN Group
c/o St. Davnet's Hospital
Monaghan

629. Mr. John Cronin
Co. Cork

630. Nursing Officers &
Deputy Nursing Officers
St. Stephen's Hospital
Co. Cork

631. National Nursing Council
SIPTU

632. Area Public Health Nurses
Western Health Board

633. Ms. Myra Sherry
Co. Kildare

634. Ms. Evelyn Conran
Dublin 14

635. Ms. Anne Moynihan
Co. Limerick

636. Ms. Bernadette Gannon
Galway

637. Nurse Teachers Group in the
Services of People with
Mental Handicap

638. Ms. Anne Cardiff
Wexford General Hospital

639. Midwives
Erinville Maternity Hospital
Cork

640. Ms. Patricia Mearley
Dublin 18

641. Outpatient Department
James Connolly Memorial Hospital
Dublin 15

642. Carlow/Kilkenny Home Care Team
St. Luke's Hospital
Kilkenny

643. Ms. Anne-Marie Lanigan
South Eastern Health Board

644. Nurses from
James Connolly Memorial Hospital
Dublin 15

645. Nursing Officer Group

646. Ms. Eithna Gaffney
& Ms. Eileen Moylan
Dublin 6W

647. Ms. Noreen Delaney
Co. Tipperary

648. Ms. Siobhan Carroll O'Brien
Co. Cork

649. Ms. Mary McMahon
Limerick Regional Hospital

650. Ms. Margaret Lally
Limerick Regional Hospital

651. Ms. Pauline Kilcoyne
Limerick Regional Hospital

652. Ms. Mary Keary
Co. Galway

653. Nursing Officers &
Deputy Nursing Officers
Louth/Meath Mental Health Services

654. Ms. Christina Hickey
Kilkenny

655. NCHD Committee
Irish Medical Organisation

656. Ms. Rosaleen Crawley Clare
Co. Louth

657. Ms. Eithne Cusack
Dublin 15

658. Ms. Olga Price

659. Mr. Paddy Hyde
Southern Health Board

660. Ms. Nuala Rafferty
Co. Meath

661. Ms. Helen O'Connor
Co. Kerry

662. Senior Staff Nurses
Renal Unit
Beaumont Hospital

663. Domiciliary Midwives

664. Ms. Rose McLoughlin
Dublin 4

665. J.C.M. Unit
James Connolly
Special Children's Hospital
Carndonagh

666. Lecturers
Department of Nursing
National University of Ireland - Cork

667. An Bord Altranais

668. Registered Nurses
College of Commerce
Cork

669. *Irish Nurses Organisation

670. Ms. Kay Coburn
Carlow

671. Group of Nurses
Forensic Services
Central Mental Hospital

672. Mr. Seamus O'Mahony
Co. Dublin

673. Nurse Managers
Letterkenny General Hospital

674. Anonymous

675. Clonmel Branch of the
Psychiatric Nurses Association

676. Temporary Nurses
North Eastern Health Board

677. P Madden
Southern Health Board

678. Public Health Nurses
Ballinasloe

679. Ms. Mary Byrne
North Eastern Health Board

680. Ms. Noreen Lyons
Co. Kerry

681. Dr. J Bernard Walsh, Dublin 8

682. Quality Assurance in
Nursing Association

683. SIPTU Forensic Psychiatric Nurses
Central Mental Hospital

684. Ms. Bernadette McGough
Co. Monaghan

685. M H Gilmartin
University College Hospital
Cork

686. Ms. Kathleen Harrington
Co. Tipperary

687. Nursing Alliance

688. Ms. Maura Tummon
Galway

689. Irish Public Health Nurses Nationwide

690. Mr. Thomas Keary
Co. Galway

691. Mr. John Shannon

*(See No: 669) This submission included submissions from the following INO Sections: A&E Special Interest Group, Practice Nurse Section, Occupational Health Nurse Section, Registered Nurse Mental Handicap Section, Nurse Tutors and Clinical Teachers Section, Midwives Section, Operating Department Nurses Section, Orthopaedic Nurses Section, Association for the Elderly, Neonatal Nurse Section. It also contained submissions from co-ordinators, degree nurses, tutors, in-service education, specialist nurses, hospital branches - individuals, public health nurses, management and ward sisters.

692. The Western Branch Institute
of Community Health Nursing

693. Anonymous

694. Mr. Patrick J McDermott
Co. Roscommon

695. Chief Executive Officers
from the Health Boards

696. C.A. MacGregor
Co. Louth

697. Ms. Rosaleen Murnane
Dublin 7

698. The Blood Transfusion Service Board

699. Community Psychiatric Nurses
Longford/Westmeath Catchment Area
Midland Health Board

700. IMPACT
The Public Sector Trade Union

701. Psychiatric Nurses Association

702. The Adelaide Hospital Society

703. The Nurse Tutors and
Clinical Teachers Section of the
Irish Nurses' Organisation

704. Monaghan Branch of the
Psychiatric Nurses Association

705. A/CNO's/Tutor in the
Mental Handicap Discipline
Eastern Health Board

706. Offshore Island based PHN's
in Co. Galway

707. Ms. Mary Fahy, Westmeath

708. Ward Sisters
University College Hospital Galway

709. Ms. Anna Monaghan
Rotunda Hospital, Dublin 7

710. Ms. Kathleen McLellan
Dublin 6

711. Ms. Mary E Doherty
Co. Donegal

712. Ms. Margaret McCafferty
Sligo General Hospital

713. Ms. Ann Gallagher
Co. Donegal

714. Ms. Katherine Croffy
Co. Galway

715. Mrs. Brigid Barron
Co. Clare

716. Ms. Una Webster
Co. Cork

717. Ms. Elizabeth Kiely
Co. Tipperary

718. Mr. David Kieran
Co. Tipperary

719. Nursing Practice
Development Co-ordinators
St. James's Hospital

720. St. James's Hospital
Dublin 8

721. Ms. Stephanie Ryan
Co. Tipperary

722. Ms. Iris O'Neill
Dublin 4

723. RNMH's
St. Vincent's Centre
Dublin 7

724. Nursing Staff
University College Hospital, Galway

725. Ms. Phil Gunning
Co. Galway

726. School of Nursing
Cork Voluntary Hospitals

727. Ms. Nuala Cashlin
Co. Donegal

728. Class 96/97 Diploma in Child
and Adolescent Psychiatric Nursing

729. Ms. Brigid Caldwell
Co. Longford

730. Ms. Mina Lalor
Co. Tipperary

731. Mr. Thomas C Keary
Co. Galway

732. Ms. Margaret Duggan
Co. Tipperary

733. Ms. Margaret Hewitt
Co. Tipperary

734. Unit Directors of Child Education
and Development Centres
Galway County Association for
Mentally Handicapped Children

735. Occupational Health Nurses
Association of Ireland (as per No: 747)

736. Public Health Nurses Section INO

737. INO Nursing Staff
St. Anne's Children's Centre
Galway

738. Ms. Denise Freiberg
Co. Tipperary

739. Education Committee Irish Practice
Nurses Association (Munster Branch)

740. Western Health Board Section INO

741. North-Western Health Board
Section INO

742. Ms. Margaret Foley-Bergin
Co. Tipperary

743. Ward Sisters
COPE Foundation, Montenotte

744. Staff Nurses
COPE Foundation, Montenotte

745. Mrs. Catherine M Flanagan
Bon Secours Hospital

746. Mr. Malachy Feely
Co. Navan

747. Occupational Health Nurses
(as per No: 735)

748. Ms. Rosemary Anne McKean
Co. Dublin

749. Nurse Tutors
Nurse Education Centre
Bon Secours Hospital

750. Susan Hurley & Breeda Daly
COPE Foundation

751. IT Nurses from St. James's,
Meath & Adelaide Hospitals

752. Irish Hospital Consultants Association

753. Nurses from
St. Patrick Community Hospital
Fermoy

754. PNA Committee
St. John of God's Psychiatric Services
Stillorgan

755. Ms. Margaret O'Keeffe
Co. Tipperary

756. Midwives Section INO

757. Ms. Maureen Caffrey
Co. Meath

758. Mr. Michael Shasby
Dublin 7

759. Barbara Fitzgerald, Mary Kelly,
Patricia Gilhooley & Sheila Fitzgerald
Participants from Workshop No: 10
Grand Hotel, Malahide

760. Ms. Ann Kelly
Co. Dublin

761. Mr. Colin Griffiths, Co. Kildare

762. Ms. Roisin Meenan
Dublin 12

763. The Royal College of Psychiatrists
- Irish Division

764. Institute of Community
Health Nursing

765. Peamount Hospital

766. Midwifery Tutors
National Maternity Hospital
Holles Street

767. The Health Board Programme
Managers Representative Group

768. Patricia Skelly, Dublin 15

769. Independent Domiciliary
Midwives of Ireland

770. The Social and
Community Care Department
Cork College of Commerce

771. Cork and Kerry
Nurse Education Committee

772. Ms. Pauline Doyle
& Ms. Heather Kevelighan
St. Vincent's Hospital, Elm Park

773. Ms. Bridget Kinsella
Co. Wexford

774. Community Nursing Staff
Brothers of Charity Services
Glanmire

775. Professor John Carroll
Dublin City University

776. Ms. Maura Nash
COPE Foundation, Montenotte

777. Ms. Nora O'Sullivan
COPE Foundation, Montenotte

778. National University of Ireland

779. Rehabilitation/Rheumatology Unit
Our Lady's Hospice
Harold's Cross

780. Dr. Seamus Cowman
Royal College of Surgeons in Ireland

781. EHB's Acute Hospitals and Services
for the Elderly Programme Committee

782. Association of Irish Nurse Managers

783. Paediatric Nurse Tutors and Clinical
Teachers from Our Lady's Hospital,
Temple Street and the National
Children's Hospital, Harcourt Street
& Director of Nursing, Our Lady's
Hospital; Crumlin.

784. Mr. Michael B Murphy
Cork University Hospital

785. Health Service Employers Agency

786. ICU Staff
St. John's Hospital, Limerick

787. Nursing Alliance

Appendix Two

List of People Whom the Commission Met

An Bord Altranais   1991 - 1997 Board
                       1997 - 2002 Board

Mr. Frank Ahern, Director of Personnel, Department of Health and Children

Ms. Ann Anglesey, Matron, St. Vincent's Hospital, Dungarvan, Co. Waterford

Ms. Sheila Armstrong, Superintendent Public Health Nurse, Eastern Health Board

Mr. Gerard Barry, Chief Executive Officer, Health Service Employers Agency

Ms. Josephine Bartley, Director of Nursing, Beaumont Hospital, Dublin

Mr. Tom Beegan, Programme Manager, South Eastern Health Board

Ms. Cecily Begley, Head of Department of Nursing Studies, Trinity College, Dublin

Dr. Michael Boland, Irish College of General Practitioners

Ms. Roisin Boland, Head of Casualty Department, The Adelaide & Meath Hospital, Dublin incorporating the National Children's Hospital

Ms. Betty Brady, Director of Nursing Studies, Dublin City University

Mr. Danny Brennan, Registrar, Letterkenny Institute of Technology

Mr. Pat Brosnan, Chief Nursing Officer, Mid-Western Health Board

Mr. Jim Brown, Director of Nursing, Letterkenny General Hospital

Mr. Stiofan de Burca, Chief Executive Officer, Mid-Western Health Board

Ms. Alice Burke, Acting Matron, General Hospital, Portlaoise

Mr. Brendan Byrne, Chief Nursing Officer, South Eastern Health Board

Mr. Eddie Byrne, Director of Nursing, Cavan General Hospital

Ms. Maureen Caffery, Co-ordinator of Services for the Elderly, North Eastern Health Board

Mr. Bernard Carey, Principal Officer, Nursing Policy Unit, Department of Health and Children

Ms. Christine Carney, Assistant General Secretary, IMPACT

Ms. Ann Carrigy, Director of Nursing, Mater Hospital, Dublin

Ms. Emer Carroll, Superintendent Public Health Nurse, South Eastern Health Board

Professor John Carroll, Registrar, Dublin City University

Ms. Johanna Cashman, Superintendent Public Health Nurse, Mid-Western Health Board

Professor George Castledine, Assistant Dean, University of England, Birmingham

Ms. Ann Clarke, Superintendent Public Health Nurse, Eastern Health Board

Ms. Jean Clarke, Lecturer/Co-ordinator Higher Diploma in Nursing Studies, Trinity College Dublin

Ms. Andy Cochrane, Clinical Teacher, Temple Street Children's Hospital, Dublin

Ms. Stasia Cody, Superintendent Public Health Nurse, Eastern Health Board

Mr. Leo Colgan, Registrar, University of Limerick

Mr. Pat Colgan, Management Consultant, Institute of Public Administration

Ms. Una Collins, Director of Nursing, Brothers of Charity, Bawnmore, Limerick

Ms. Sarah Condell, Principal Nurse Tutor, The Adelaide & Meath Hospital, Dublin Incorporating the National Children's Hospital

Ms. Grainne Connolly, Head of Change Management Unit, Health Service Employers Agency

Ms. Maura Connolly, Matron, National Children's Hospital (The Adelaide & Meath Hospital, Dublin incorporating the National Children's Hospital)

Ms. Juliette Cotter, Practice Nurse, Kinsale, Co. Cork

Ms. Mary Courtney, Director of Nursing, Portiuncula Hospital, Ballinasloe, Co. Galway

Mr. Martin Cowley, Chief Executive Officer, Mater Hospital, Dublin

Mr. James Coyle, Registrar, Athlone Institute of Technology

Ms. Katherine Craughwell, Director of Nursing/Services Development, North-Western Health Board

Ms. Mary Cronin, Independent Domiciliary Midwives of Ireland

Ms. Nora Cummins, Superintendent Public Health Nurse, Eastern Health Board

Ms. Mary Curran, Superintendent Public Health Nurse, North Western Health Board

Ms. Kathleen Curry, Superintendent Public Health Nurse, North Eastern Health Board

Ms. Chris Daly, Matron, St. Camillus' Hospital, Limerick

Ms. Margaret Daly, Superintendent Public Health Nurse, Southern Health Board

Ms. Ann Doherty, Matron, Clonakilty Hospital, Co. Cork

Ms. Una Doherty, Superintendent Public Health Nurse, South Eastern Health Board

Ms. Mary Dolan, Chief Nursing Officer, North Eastern Health Board

Ms. Marie Dooley, Superintendent Public Health Nurse, North Eastern Health Board

Mr. James Doran, Head of Industrial Relations, Health Service Employers Agency

Mr. Liam Doran, General Secretary Designate, Irish Nurses Organisation

Ms. Eleanor Dowling, Superintendent Public Health Nurse, Midland Health Board

Ms. Pauline Doyle, Director of Nursing, St. Vincent's Hospital, Elm Park

Ms. Mary Duff, Director of Nursing, Our Lady of Lourdes Hospital, Drogheda

Ms. Maeve Dwyer, Matron, National Maternity Hospital, Holles St., Dublin

Ms. Grace Faher, Superintendent Public Health Nurse, Eastern Health Board

Mr. Martin Farrell, Chief Nursing Officer, Eastern Health Board

Mr. Bernard Finnegan, Matron, Wexford General Hospital

Ms. Siobhan Finnegan, Head of Department of Nursing Studies, Athlone Institute of Technology

Ms. Catherine Fitzgibbon, Superintendent Public Health Nurse, Western Health Board

Ms. Margaret Fitzpatrick, Superintendent Public Health Nurse, Eastern Health Board

Ms. Nora Fitzpatrick, Director of Nursing, Limerick Regional Hospital Group

Mr. P.J. Fitzpatrick, Chief Executive Officer, Eastern Health Board

Ms. Helen Flint, Director of Nursing Research and Development, Eastern Health Board

Ms. Ann Flynn, Superintendent Public Health Nurse, Eastern Health Board

Mr. Matt Flynn, Director of Nursing, Cregg House, Sligo

Mr. Bill Frewen, Chief Nursing Officer, South-Eastern Health Board

Mr. Joe Gallagher, Chief Nursing Officer, North Western Health Board

Ms. Elva Gannon, Head of Employers Advisory Service, Health Service Employers Agency

Ms. Rosa Gardiner, Superintendent Public Health Nurse, South Eastern Health Board

Ms. Barbara Garrigan, Principal Nurse Tutor, St. James's Hospital, Dublin

Mr. Pat Gaughan, Programme Manager, North Western Health Board

Ms. Mary Gobbi, Associate Researcher, Nurse Education and Training Education, Project (NEATE)

Mr. John Griffin, Principal Nurse, Cregg House, Sligo

Ms. Anne Gunning, Director of Community Nursing Services, St. John of God, Stillorgan

Ms. Attracta Halpin, Assistant Registrar, National University of Ireland

Ms. Christine Hancock, General Secretary, Royal College of Nursing, London

Mr. Eamon Hannan, Former Chief Executive Officer, Western Health Board

Sr. Triona Harvey, Department of Nursing, National University of Ireland - Dublin

Ms. Breda Hayes, Director of Nursing Services for the Elderly, Eastern Health Board

Mr. Bernie Heddigan, Programme Manager, Western Health Board

Ms. Christine Hickey, Association of Community Psychiatric Nurses

Ms. Judith Hill, Chief Nursing Officer, Department of Health and Social Services, Northern Ireland

Ms. Mairead Hogan, Director of Nursing, Longford/Westmeath General Hospital, Mullingar

Mr. Tom Houlihan, Chief Nursing Officer, St. Vincent's Hospital, Fairview, Dublin

Ms. Bridget Howley, Director of Nursing, University College Hospital, Galway

Ms. Geralyn Hynes, Practice Nurse, Dublin

Irish Nurses Organisation, Representatives of Nurse Tutors Section

Mr. Nicholas Jermyn, Chief Executive Officer, St. Vincent's Hospital, Elm Park, Dublin

Ms. Colette Kearney, Editor, Aersceala, Aer Lingus

Sr. Antoinette Kelliher, Principal Nurse Tutor, Our Lady's Hospital for Sick Children, Crumlin

Ms. Mary Kelly, Director of Nursing, Rotunda Hospital, Dublin

Ms. Mary Kilmartin, Deputy Director of Nursing, University College Hospital, Cork

Ms. Breege Kirby, Practice Nurse, Health Centre, Carndonagh, Co. Donegal

Ms. Veronica Kow, Nurse Tutor, Our Lady's Hospital for Sick Children, Crumlin

Mr. Roy Lane, Director of Nursing, General Hospital Tullamore

Ms. Mai Lanigan, Former Director of Nursing, Waterford Regional Hospital

Ms. Patricia Leahy-Warren, Public Health Nurse, Southern Health Board

Ms. Catherine Leavy, Superintendent Public Health Nurse, Midland Health Board

Ms. Josephine Leyden, Principal Nurse Tutor, James Connolly Memorial Hospital, Blanchardstown

Ms. Mary Liston, Superintendent Public Health Nurse, Mid-Western Health Board

Ms. Emily Logan, Director of Nursing, Our Lady's Hospital for Sick Children, Crumlin

Mr. Gareth Long, Deputy Director, NEATE Project

Mr. Pat Lynch, Higher Executive Officer, Information Management Unit, Department of Health and Children

Mr. Pat Lyons, Chief Executive Officer, Beaumont Hospital

Mr. Hugh Magee, Statistician, Department of Health and Children

Ms. Aileen Maguire, Director of Nursing, Louth/Meath General Hospital, Dundalk

Ms. Mary Mahon, Superintendent Public Health Nurse, South Eastern Health Board

Professor Dermot McAleese, Chairperson, Commission on Public Service Pensions

Ms. Ann McCarthy, Assistant Director of Nursing, Regional Maternity Hospital, Limerick

Ms. Mary McCarthy, Director of Nursing, The Adelaide & Meath Hospital, Dublin
Incorporating the National Children's Hospital

Dr. David McCutcheon, Chief Executive Officer, The Adelaide & Meath Hospital, Dublin
Incorporating the National Children's Hospital

Ms. Joan McDermott, D'Alton Home, Claremorris, Co. Mayo

Ms. Lena McDermott, Unit Nursing Officer, Our Lady's Hospital for Sick Children, Crumlin

Ms. Mary McDermott, Superintendent Public Health Nurse, Western Health Board

Mr. Oliver McDonagh, National Nursing Official, SIPTU

Mr. John McEvoy, Secretary, Central Applications Office, Galway

Mr. George McFadden, Head of Department of Nursing Studies, Letterkenny Institute of Technology

Mr. Conor McGinn, Secretary, Commission on Public Service Pensions

Ms. Maria McInerney, Midwifery Tutor, Regional Maternity Hospital, Limerick

Mr. Jarlath McKenna, Head of Department of Nursing Studies, Waterford Institute of Technology

Mr. Peter McKenna, Association of Community Psychiatric Nurses

Ms. Brid McLoughlin, Aras Mathair Pol, Castlerea, Co. Galway

Ms. Cliodhna McLoughlin, Independent Domiciliary Midwives of Ireland

Mr. Stephen McManus, Registrar, Dundalk Institute of Technology

Ms. Maureen McNulty, Marymount Nursing Home, Lucan

Ms. Wilma McPherson, Director of Nursing, St. Thomas and Guy's Hospital, London

Ms. Geraldine McSweeney, Principal Nurse Tutor, St. Vincent's Hospital, Elm Park, Dublin

Medical Organisations - Representatives from the following:

Irish College of General Practitioners
Irish Hospital Consultants Association
Irish Medical Organisation
Medical Council
Royal College of Physicians of Ireland
Royal College of Psychiatrists - Irish Division
Royal College of Surgeons in Ireland

Sr. Pius Meehan, Director of Nursing, St. Luke's Hospital, Kilkenny

Mr. Tom Meehan, Lecturer, Queensland University of Technology

Mr. Padraic Mellet, Higher Education Authority

Ms. Sally Miller, Independent Domiciliary Midwives of Ireland

Ms. Maria Molloy, Superintendent Public Health Nurse, Mid-Western Health Board

Mr. Sean Molloy, Chief Nursing Officer, St. Loman's Hospital, Dublin

Ms. Gertie Monagle, Matron, Carndonagh District Hospital, Co. Donegal

Professor M.A. Moran, Registrar, University College Cork

Ms. Marian Moutray, School of Nursing and Midwifery, Queen's University, Belfast

Ms. Nora Mulcahy, Head of Department of Nursing, University of Limerick

Mr. Gerry Mulholland, Director of Nursing, Stewarts Hospital, Palmerstown

Ms. Catherine Murphy, Communications Officer, Southern Health Board

Ms. Cathy Murphy, Head of Department of Nursing, National University of Ireland - Galway

Mr. Seamus Murphy, Industrial Relations Officer, Psychiatric Nurses Association

Ms. Maura Nash, Director of Nursing, COPE Foundation, Cork

Mr. Martin Newell, Manager, Central Applications Office, Galway

Mr. John Nolan, Registrar, National University of Ireland

Mr. John O' Brien, Chief Executive Officer, St. James' Hospital, Dublin

Ms. Mary O' Brien, Director of Nursing, Erinville Hospital, Cork

Mr. Jim O' Callaghan, Head of Dept of Nursing Studies, St. Angela's College, Sligo

Mr. Brian O' Connell, Internal Communications Officer, Aer Lingus

Ms. Rhona O' Connell, Midwifery Tutor, St. Finbarr's/Erinville Hospitals, Cork

Ms. Ann O' Connor, Superintendent Public Health Nurse, Southern Health Board

Ms. Irene O'Connor, Matron, St. Ita's Hospital, Newcastlewest, Co. Limerick

Ms. Ita O' Dwyer, Director of Nursing, Coombe Women's Hospital, Dublin

Dr. Fergus O' Ferrall, Director of Adelaide Hospital Society, Dublin

Ms. Sheila O' Kelly, Barrister-at-Law

Ms. Sheila O' Malley, Superintendent Public Health Nurse, Eastern Health Board

Professor I. O' Muircheartaigh, Registrar, National University of Ireland - Galway

Ms. Dolores O' Neill, Superintendent Public Health Nurse, Western Health Board

Ms. Joan O' Neill, Director of Nursing, Leopardstown Park Hospital

Ms. Margaret O' Regan, Superintendent Public Health Nurse, Southern Health Board

Ms. Peig O' Riordan, Acting Ward Sister, Mercy Hospital, Cork

Mr. Donal O' Shea, Chief Executive Officer, North Eastern Health Board

Ms. Rita O' Shea, Director of Nursing, Temple Street Children's Hospital, Dublin

Ms. Kay O' Sullivan, Director of Nursing, University College Hospital, Cork

Ms. Marion O' Sullivan, National Council for Educational Awards

Ms. Patrice O' Sullivan, Principal Nurse Tutor, Mater Hospital, Dublin

Ms. Breda Power, Superintendent Public Health Nurse, Southern Health Board

Mr. Liam Power, Director of Nursing Services, Peamount, Newcastle, Co. Dublin

Mr. Robert Quinn, Director of Nursing, St. Joseph's Hospital, Clonmel

Representatives from those in Mental Handicap Nursing who forwarded written submissions to the Commission
Representative Group of all Grades of Staff from St. Joseph's Hospital, Clonsilla
Representative Group of all Grades of Staff from Stewarts Hospital, Palmerstown

Ms. Susan Reilly, Assistant Principal Officer, Nursing Policy Unit, Department of Health and Children

Mr. Paul Robinson, Deputy Chief Executive Officer, Mid-Western Health Board

Sr. Laurentia Roche, Director of Nursing, Mercy Hospital, Cork

Ms. Johanna Ronan, Barrister-at-Law

Ms. Anne-Marie Ryan, Principal Nurse Tutor, Beaumont Hospital

Ms. Rosemary Ryan, Director of Nursing, St. James's Hospital, Dublin

Ms. Sheelagh Ryan, Chief Executive Officer, Western Health Board

Ms. Sheila Ryan, Director of Services, St. Vincent's, Lisnagry, Co. Limerick

Ms. Ellen Savage, Lecturer, Department of Nursing, National University of Ireland - Cork

Ms. Teresa Scully, Superintendent Public Health Nurse, Eastern Health Board

Ms. Deirdre Seery, Matron., Cottage Hospital, Drogheda, Co. Louth

Mr. Michael Shasby, ACNO, Dept. of Psychiatry and Old Age, Eccles St., Dublin

Ms. Katherine Sheeran, Director of Nursing, James Connolly Memorial Hospital, Blanchardstown

Ms. Ann Sheridan, Principal Nurse Tutor, St. John of God, Stillorgan

Professor Helen Simons, Director of NEATE Project

Dr. Oliver Slevin, Chief Executive Officer, National Board for Nursing, Midwifery and Health Visiting for Northern Ireland

Ms. Aideen Stanley, Caiseal Geal Nursing Home, Castlegar, Galway

Student Nurses and Recently Qualified Staff Nurses from St. James's Hospital, Dublin

Student Nurses from St. Joseph's Hospital, Clonsilla

Student Nurses from Stewarts Hospital, Palmerstown

Ms. Helen Thornton, Superintendent Public Health Nurse, North Eastern Health Board

Ms. Josephine Tiernan, Director of Nursing, Mayo General Hospital

Mr. Mark Tyrrell, Lecturer, Department of Nursing, National University of Ireland - Cork

Ms. Celine Walsh, Superintendent Public Health Nurse, Eastern Health Board

Mr. Manus Ward, Chief Executive Officer, North Western Health Board

Ms. Eileen Weir, Superintendent Public Health Nurse, Eastern Health Board

Ms. Joan Wilmot, Director of Nursing, Royal Hospital, Donnybrook

Ms. Maureen Windle, Programme Manager, Eastern Health Board

Mr. Tim Wray, Head of Internal Communications, Telecom Eireann

Dr. Margo Wrigley, Royal College of Psychiatry - Irish Division

Appendix Three

List of People Whom the Commission Met During the Visit to Australia

16th March '98	Chief Nurses	
Judith Meppem	Chief Nursing Officer	Health Department NSW.
David White	Chief Nurse	South Australia Health Commission
Sue Norrie	Principle Nursing Advisor	Health Advisory Unit, Queensland
Suzanne Williams	Chief Nursing Officer	Department of Health Western Australia
Verity Bondfield	Chief Nurse	Department of ACT Health & Community Care
Zoe Cuthbert	Chief Nurse	Tasmanian Department of Community & H.S.
Kathleen McLauglin	Chief Nurse	Department of Human Resources, Victoria
Frances Hughes	Chief Advisor (Nursing)	Ministry of Health, New Zealand
Colleen Singleton	Chief Executive Officer	Nursing Council of New Zealand
Judy Kilpatrick	Chairperson	Nursing Council of New Zealand
Jenny Carryer	Chief Executive	New Zealand, College of Nursing
Kerry Russell	Associate Director	Health Department, Nursing Branch NSW

16th March '98	Area Directors of Nursing	
Jenny Becker	Area Director of Nursing	Central Coast Area Health Service NSW
Joan Englert	Area Director of Nursing	Central Sydney Area Health Service NSW
Val Coughlin-West	Area Director of Nursing	Hunter Area Health Service NSW
Jan Stow	Director of Clinical Services	Westmeath Hospital
Jenny Kidd	DON & Patient Care Services	St. Vincent's Hospital
Patricia Tyson	Director of Nursing	Nepean Health, NSW.
Rosemary Snodgrass	Director of Nursing	New South Wales RNSH
Wilna Taylor	Area Director of Nursing	Mid Northern Coast Health Service NSW
Irene Jones	Area Director of Nursing	Midwestern Health Service NSW

Jean Shelley	Area Director of Nursing	Southern Health Service NSW
Rosemary Cullen	Policy Analyst	Special Projects, Nursing Branch NSW
Lisa Wagg	Project Officer	Health Department, Nursing Branch NSW
Julie Williams	Careers Advisor	Health Department, Nursing Branch NSW
Ann O'Donoghue	Acting Professional Advisor	Health Department, RNA Nursing Branch

17th March 1998   *Council of Deans of Nursing*

Professor Peter Sheehan	Vice Chancellor	Australian Catholic University, Sydney
Prof. E. Cameron-Traub	Dean Faculty of Health Science	Australian Catholic University, Sydney
Professor M. McMillan	Dean Faculty of Nursing	University of Newcastle, NSW
Ms. Bronwyn Jones	Department of Nursing	Edith Conway University
Ass. Prof. Pauline Nugent	Head, School of Nursing	Deakin University, Burwood, Victoria
Ms. Roslyn Reilly	Head, Department of Nursing	University of Southern Queensland
Ms. Gwen Behrens	Department of Nursing	Avondale College
Professor Jill White	Dean Faculty of Nursing	University of Technology, Sydney.
Professor Lynette Russell	Dean Faculty of Nursing	The University of Sydney
Ms. Colleen Singleton	Chief Executive Officer	Nursing Council of New Zealand
Ms. Judy Kirkpatrick	Chair	Nursing Council of New Zealand

17th March 1998   *Nursing Council NSW*

Jan Dent	Executive Director	Nurses Registration Board NSW
Michael Cleary	Associate Executive Director	Nurses Registration Board NSW
Joan Englert	President	Nurses Registration Board NSW
Rosemary Snodgrass	Deputy President	Nurses Registration Board NSW
Marlyn Gendek	Acting Chief Executive Officer	Australian Nursing Council Inc.
Wanda Lawler	Registrar	ACT Registration Board
Colleen Singleton	Chief Executive Officer	New Zealand Nursing Council
Judy Kilpatrick	Chairperson	New Zealand Nursing Council
Loraine Ferguson	Acting Executive Officer	NSW College of Nursing
Jill Lliffe	Manager Professional Services	NSW Nurses' Association

18th March 1998	Faculty of Nursing, University of Newcastle	
Professor Helen Baker	Professor Clinical Nursing Research	University of Newcastle, NSW
Dr. Diana Keatinge	Associate Prof. Clinical Nursing Research	University of Newcastle, NSW
Margaret McEniery	Assistant Dean, Course Work Programme	University of Newcastle, NSW
Liz Bujack	Assistant Dean, Midwifery Programme	University of Newcastle, NSW
Professor Irene Madjar	Assistant Dean, Postgraduate Research	University of Newcastle, NSW
Ann Williams	Assistant Dean, Undergraduate Programme	University of Newcastle, NSW
Shirley Schulz-Robinson	Senior Lecturer	University of Newcastle, NSW
Terrence McCann	Lecturer	University of Newcastle, NSW
18th March 1998	John Hunter Hospital	
Nerida Ambler	Manager Nurse Education	John Hunter Hospital, Newcastle, NSW
Elizabeth Day	Acting Director of Nursing, Medicine	John Hunter Hospital, Newcastle NSW
Healther Chislett	Acting DON, Surgical Services + ICU	John Hunter Hospital, Newcastle, NSW
Anne Saxton	DON Obstetrics & Gynaecology	John Hunter Hospital, Newcastle, NSW
Rosalie Shaw	CNC Obstetrics & Gynaecology	John Hunter Hospital, Newcastle, NSW
Jennina Porter	NUM - ICU + Clinical Nurse Associate	John Hunter Hospital, Newcastle, NSW
Kate Rawlings	DON, Executive Officer CAYNet	John Hunter Hospital, Newcastle, NSW
Carol Joans	Perioperative CNS/Clinical Nurse Associate	John Hunter Hospital, Newcastle, NSW
19th March 1998	University of Technology Sydney	
Prof. Christine Duffield	Assistant Dean Post Graduate Programmes	Faculty of Nursing.
19th March 1998	Royal Alexandra, New Children's Hospital, Parramatta	
Jan Minnis	Director of Nursing	New Children's Hospital
Margaret Bunker	Deputy Director of Nursing	New Children's Hospital
Kaye Spence	Clinical Nurse Consultant, Neonatology	New Children's Hospital
Lyn Brodie	Nurse Unit Manager, Neonatal ITU	New Children's Hospital
Glenys Amy	Senior Nurse Educator	New Children's Hospital
Libba O'Riordan	Clinical Nurse Consultant, Oncology	New Children's Hospital

Karen Rankin	Nurse Unit Manager, Isolation	New Children's Hospital
Cecila Lau Phd	Nursing Information and Clinical Carepaths	New Children's Hospital
Jane Gregurke	Nurse Unit Manager, Paediatric ICU	New Children's Hospital
Helen Giles	Nurse Unit Manager, A & E.	New Children's Hospital
Jeanette Flanagan	Operating Theatre, Nurse Unit Manager	New Children's Hospital
Professor Sue Nagy	Paediatric Nursing, Hospital Academic	New Children's Hospital
20th March 1998	**Central Sydney Area Health Services**	
Dr. Diana Horvath	Chief Executive Officer	Central Sydney Area Health Services
Joan Englert	Area Director Nursing Services	Central Sydney Area Health Services
Ann Kelly	Director of Nursing & Nurse Co-ordinator	Balmain Hospital, CSAHS
Bernadette Loughnane	Nurse Co-ordinator Neuroscience's Group	Royal Prince Alfred Hospital, CSAHS
Vicki Hathaway	Director of Nursing	Canterbury Hospital, CSAHS.
Jocelyn McLean	Case Manager, Thoracic Surgery	Royal Prince Alfred Hospital, CSAHS
Mai Blane	Best Practice Co-ordinator, Cl. Path Project	Royal Prince Alfred Hospital, CSAHS
Robyn White	DON, Nurse Co-ordinator Community	Central Sydney Area Health Services
Margaret Murphy	CNC, Emergency Department	Royal Prince Alfred Hospital, CSAHS
Natalie McKenzie	Acting Clinical Nurse Consultant, ICU	Royal Prince Alfred Hospital, CSAHS
Lynne Fairservice	Clinical Educator ICU	Royal Prince Alfred Hospital, CSAHS
Pauline Green	CNC, Midwifery Parent Ed.	Royal Prince Alfred Hospital, CSAHS
Gary Rowley	DON Nurse Co-ordinator Mental Health	Rozelle Hospital, CSAHS
Kerry Russell	Director of Nursing	Concord Hospital, CSAHS
23rd March 1998	**Embassy of Ireland**	
Mr. Pat Bourne	First Secretary	Embassy of Ireland, Canberra, ACT
Mr. Joe Sheehan	Third Secretary	Embassy of Ireland, Canberra, ACT

23rd March 1998	*Royal College of Nursing, Australia*	
Elizabeth Foley	Professional Programmes Manager	Royal College of Nursing, Canberra
Julie Spensor	Education Programme Manager	Royal College of Nursing, Canberra
Jeanann Rommage	Co-ordinator of College Societies	Royal College of Nursing, Canberra

23rd March 1998	*Commonwealth Department of Health and Family Services (DOHFS)*	
Patrick Colmer	Director Health Workforce Unit	DOHFS
Therese Mansen	Health Workforce Unit	DOHFS
Heather Martin	Royal College of Nursing	

23rd March 1998	*Department of Employment, Education, Training and Youth Affairs (DEETYA)*	
Peggy Spratt	Assistant Director	Ed. Developments/ International Section
Alan Ford	Higher Education	DEETYA

Appendix Four

Quarterly National Household Survey September - November 1997 - Module on Nursing Care

Questionnaire

This module was asked only where the person's age was 18 or over and where the person was being interviewed directly. The answers were recorded on laptop computers using Computer-Assisted Personnel Interview (CAPI) software.

1. Have you had personal contact with nursing services within the past two years?
    This could be either as a patient or visiting or accompanying a patient.

    YES/NO

    If NO, ask no more questions from this module.

    If YES, display this prompt and ask Q2:

    "I would now like you to consider the most important contact you had with nurses delivering health care in the past 2 years. I will ask you some questions about this contact."

2. On that occasion, were you...

    (a) A patient

    (b) Next of kin of a patient

    (c) Other

3. Where was this contact with nursing services?

    (a) In a hospital

    (b) In the community

    (c) In you own home or a relative's home

    (d) In a nursing home

    (e) Other

4. If Q2 is (a) ask questions 4a1 - 4a8:

    "On that occasion, how would you rate the following aspects of the nursing service that you received as a patient? Please indicate whether you consider the nursing service on that occasion as Poor, Adequate, Good, or Excellent or if the particular question is Not Relevant to you."

    (For each question, the PC will display the 5 response categories.)

    4a1: Attitude to you:
    4a2: Time spent with you:
    4a3: Attention given in listening to you:
    4a4: Information given to you about your treatment, condition or illness:
    4a5: Instruction about your care:
    4a6: Attention given in responding to your requests for help:
    4a7: Performance of professional tasks:
    4a8: Consideration of your opinion or decisions:

Now skip to question 5.

If Q2 is (b) ask questions 4b1 - 4b4:

"On that occasion, how would you rate the following aspects of the nursing service? Please indicate whether you consider the nursing service on that occasion as Poor, Adequate, Good, or Excellent or if the particular question is Not Relevant to you."

(For each question, the PC will display the 5 response categories.)

4b1 Courtesy shown to you (general attitude, time spent with you, ability to listen):
4b2 Information given to you about the patient's condition and care:
4b3 Performance of professional tasks:
4b4 Consideration of your opinion or decisions:

Ask question 5 of all persons who answered YES to question 1.

5. Overall, what is your general rating of the nursing services given on the occasion we have been speaking about:

Poor/Adequate/Good/Excellent?

Note: Only the above 4 categories are allowed for question 5.

Appendix Five

CENTRAL STATISTICS OFFICE

Quarterly National Household Survey September-November 1997
Results of Module on Nursing Services

Main Findings.

- Over 42% of the population aged 18 or over had some contact with nursing services in the previous two years.

- Almost a quarter of the adult population had contact with nursing services as a patient in the previous two years.

- A greater proportion of women than men had some contact with nursing services, 48% of women as against 36% of men.

- Overall satisfaction with nursing services was high, with 56% giving an overall rating of "Excellent" and 34% "Good".

- Patients gave a high rating to each aspect of nursing care. The highest rating was given to nurses' Performance of Professional Tasks, rated "Good" or "Excellent" by over 90% of patients.

Methodology

The September-November 1997 quarter of the Quarterly National Household Survey (QNHS) included a number of questions designed to measure the public's level of contact with and their assessment of nursing services. The QNHS is a continuous survey covering a sample of 3,000 households per week or 39,000 per quarter. The survey began in September 1997 and a total of 33,500 households was included in the first quarter.

The questions on nursing were put to all persons aged 18 or over who were being interviewed directly. Proxy responses were not allowed, as the questions involved individual assessment of nursing services. The sample results on nursing were based on responses given directly by over 51,000 individual respondents. These were re-weighted to represent the overall population profile by sex, age group and region in April 1997, which corrects for any under- or over-representation of demographic subgroups in the results for direct respondents. The results are representative of the population aged 18 years or over resident in private households.

The questions on nursing services concerned:

- Contact with nursing services in the past two years
- Type and place of contact
- Assessment by patient of eight aspects of nursing care
- Assessment by next of kin of four aspects of nursing care
- Overall assessment of nursing services.

More details of these questions are given in Appendix 4. The results are presented in the form of percentage distributions in tables 1 to 6.

Questions 1 and 2 - Extent and Type of Contact.

Over 42% of the population aged 18 or over had some contact with nursing services in the previous two years. See table 1.

Overall, slightly more than half of those who had contact with nursing services were patients, about a third were next of kin and about 11% had contact in another capacity. See table 1.

References, Bibliography, Appendices and Acknowledgements

Table 1	Percentage of persons aged 18 years or over who had contact with nursing services in the past two years			%
			Type of Contact	
Sex	% who had contact	Patient	Next of kin	Other
Male	36.1	19.0	13.1	4.1
Female	47.9	26.8	15.6	5.6
All persons	**42.2**	**23.0**	**14.4**	**4.8**

In general, contact with nursing services is higher with increasing age. However, relatively higher percentages of women aged 25 to 39 had contact with nursing services as patients. This is probably contact with maternity services. Men in the corresponding age groups had high levels of contact with nursing services as next of kin. See table 2.

Table 2	Percentage of persons aged 18 years or over who had contact with nursing services in the past two years, classified by detailed age categories				%
				Type of contact	
Sex	Age group	% who had contact	Patient	Next of kin	Other
Male	18-19	17.7	11.7	3.3	2.7
	20-24	22.7	13.2	5.1	4.3
	25-29	33.4	14.6	14.2	4.6
	30-34	42.8	14.6	23.6	4.7
	35-39	41.7	14.1	23.0	4.6
	40-44	38.2	14.2	19.0	5.0
	45-49	36.7	16.5	16.5	3.7
	50-54	34.6	18.1	12.3	4.2
	55-59	35.4	23.2	7.8	4.4
	60-64	36.5	26.7	6.5	3.3
	65-69	42.9	32.5	6.9	3.5
	70-74	46.4	37.0	6.8	2.6
	75-79	48.9	39.2	6.9	2.8
	80-84	51.9	43.7	7.1	1.1
	85+	52.0	43.1	7.2	1.7
Total Male		**36.1**	**19.0**	**13.1**	**4.1**

Table 2 *Percentage of persons aged 18 years or over who had contact with nursing services in the past two years, classified by detailed age categories* %

Sex	Age group	% who had contact	Type of contact		
			Patient	Next of kin	Other
Female	18-19	27.4	15.8	6.0	5.6
	20-24	36.9	22.4	7.5	7.0
	25-29	50.7	32.4	12.1	6.3
	30-34	60.7	36.4	18.8	5.5
	35-39	56.1	28.1	23.1	4.9
	40-44	50.0	19.3	24.0	6.7
	45-49	48.6	19.4	23.4	5.8
	50-54	46.9	22.0	19.2	5.7
	55-59	44.0	21.5	16.5	6.0
	60-64	42.8	24.2	13.9	4.7
	65-69	45.2	26.3	13.8	5.2
	70-74	46.2	31.0	11.2	3.9
	75-79	51.5	38.5	9.4	3.6
	80-84	52.7	42.6	6.3	3.9
	85+	53.8	49.4	2.8	1.6
Total Female		**47.9**	**26.8**	**15.6**	**5.6**
Male + Female		**42.2**	**23.0**	**14.4**	**4.8**

Question 3 - Place of Contact

The details of type and place of contact and the questions on the assessment of nursing care related to the most important contact the respondent had with nurses delivering health care. Understandably, therefore, most of the replies related to hospital stays or hospital visits.

More than 90% of respondents' contact with nursing services took place in hospitals, with only very small percentages reporting contact elsewhere (in the community, in the home, in a nursing home etc.). See table 3.

The results include only a very small proportion of respondents who had contact with nursing services in a nursing home. This is because the QNHS covers private households only and does not include the resident population of nursing homes.

Table 3 Place and type of contact with nursing services						%
	Hospital	Community	Home	Nursing Home	Other	Total
Patients	93.9	2.2	2.8	0.2	1.0	100.0
Next of kin	90.2	2.3	4.8	2.5	0.3	100.0
Others	83.8	5.3	3.4	5.4	2.2	100.0
Total	**91.5**	**2.6**	**3.5**	**1.6**	**0.9**	**100.0**

Questions 4A1 to 4A8 - Patients' Assessment

The general pattern for each of these questions was for 80% or more of patients to rate the nursing services as "Good" or "Excellent". The highest "Excellent" ratings, over 50%, were in respect of *Attitude to the Patient and Performance of Professional Tasks*. See table 4.

In general, the percentages rating an aspect of nursing care as either "Poor" or "Adequate" were small. The weakest areas were *Time Spent*, rated "Poor" or Adequate" by 17% and *Information Given* (14%).

For some of the questions, a fairly high proportion considered the relevant aspect of nursing care "not relevant" (8.2% in the case of *Responding to Requests* and 11.3% in respect of *Consideration of Your Opinion*). This indicates that patients may have different expectations in relation to the different aspects of nursing care.

Table 4 Assessment made by patients of each aspect of nursing services							%
Question		Poor	Adequate	Good	Excellent	Not relevant	Total
4A1	Attitude	2.8	5.3	38.4	53.2	0.3	100.0
4A2	Time spent	4.9	12.1	39.7	41.4	1.9	100.0
4A3	Listening	4.5	8.2	40.8	44.1	2.5	100.0
4A4	Information given	5.9	8.0	37.2	43.3	5.6	100.0
4A5	Instruction about care	4.7	7.3	39.3	42.9	5.8	100.0
4A6	Response to requests	4.3	6.3	38.0	43.2	8.2	100.0
4A7	Performance of tasks	2.0	4.3	37.7	55.1	0.9	100.0
4A8	Consideration of opinion	4.0	5.9	38.7	40.2	11.3	100.0

Again, high ratings were given all round with over 85% considering the Courtesy shown to them and Performance of Professional Tasks to be "Good" or "Excellent". Over 50% rated these as "Excellent".

However, 15% of next of kin considered the Information Given about the patient's care or condition to be "Poor" or "Adequate" and over 10% gave a similar low rating to the Courtesy shown to them and Consideration of their opinion.

A smaller percentage (65.8%) rated the Consideration of their Opinion as "Good" or "Excellent". However, many next of kin (23%) did not think this point was relevant to them. See Table 5.

Table 5	Assessment made by Next of Kin of aspects of nursing care						%
		Poor	Adequate	Good	Excellent	Not relevant	Total
Question							
4B1	Courtesy	3.7	6.5	34.5	51.6	3.6	100.0
4B2	Information given	7.0	8.2	34.9	41.6	8.3	100.0
4B3	Performance of tasks	3.4	5.6	35.0	52.1	3.9	100.0
4B4	Consideration of your opinion	5.5	5.8	30.5	35.3	23.0	100.0

Question 5 - Overall Rating

This question covered all persons who had contact with nursing services in the previous two years, 56% of whom gave an overall rating of "Excellent" and 34.4% as "Good". Overall, therefore, over 90% of those aged 18 or over who had contact with nursing services in the previous two years considered the service to be "Good" or "Excellent".

On the other hand, just under 10% gave a negative assessment, 3.4% rating the quality of nursing services as "Poor" and 6.1% as just "Adequate".

The pattern of respondents' overall assessment of nursing services was similar for males and females and for the different types and places of contact with nursing. See table 6.

Table 6 *Overall assessment of nursing services* %

		Poor	Adequate	Good	Excellent	Total
Sex	Male	2.5	5.5	36.8	55.2	100.0
	Female	4.1	6.6	32.7	56.7	100.0
Type of contact	Patients	3.1	5.6	33.6	57.7	100.0
	Next of kin	4.2	6.5	34.1	55.2	100.0
	Other	3.0	7.5	38.7	50.8	100.0
Place of contact	In a hospital	3.4	6.1	34.4	56.2	100.0
	In the community	4.3	6.7	37.8	51.2	100.0
	In the home	3.8	6.3	32.3	57.6	100.0
	In a nursing home	4.1	6.3	32.3	57.3	100.0
	Other	3.1	12.3	36.8	47.9	100.0
Total		**3.4**	**6.1**	**34.4**	**56.0**	**100.0**

Acknowledgements

The Commission wishes to thank all who attended workshops and seminars during the consultative fora with a special thanks to those who facilitated/chaired workshops or who acted as rapporteurs for these meetings.

The Commission wishes to acknowledge the invaluable assistance of the following people:

Aidan Beatty and Staff, Library and Information Unit, Department of Health and Children

Sean Creedon, Telecom Eireann

Paddie Delaney, Department of Health and Social Services, Northern Ireland

John Doherty, Irish Business and Employers Confederation

Vivian Gorman, Health Research Board

John Hayden, Higher Education Authority

Muriel Heire and Staff, Library, Irish Nurses Organisation

Mary Kerr, Higher Education Authority

Pat Lynch, Information Management Unit, Department of Health and Children

Staff of the Nursing Policy Unit, Department of Health and Children

Yvonne O' Shea, Chief Education Officer, An Bord Altranais

Catherine Rooney and Staff, Library, An Bord Altranais

Staff of the Blood Policy Unit, Department of Health and Children

Brian Stout, Queen's University, Belfast

Joe Treacy, Senior Statistician, Central Statistics Office, Cork

The Commission finally wishes to record its thanks to all who gave of their time and expertise in any way which greatly assisted the Commission in its deliberations.

Wt. P60012. 5,000. 9/98. Cahill. (M29073). G.Spl.